Henry
Miller

Survival Analysis
A Practical Approach

Survival Analysis
A Practical Approach

MAHESH K.B. PARMAR AND
DAVID MACHIN
Medical Research Council Cancer Trials Office,
Cambridge, UK

JOHN WILEY & SONS
Chichester · New York · Brisbane · Toronto · Singapore

Other Wiley Editorial Offices

John Wiley & Sons, Inc., 605 Third Avenue,
New York, NY 10158-0012, USA

Jacaranda Wiley Ltd, 33 Park Road, Milton,
Queensland 4064, Australia

John Wiley & Sons (Canada) Ltd, 22 Worcester Road,
Rexdale, Ontario M9W 1L1, Canada

John Wiley & Sons (SEA) Pte Ltd, 37 Jalan Pemimpin #05-04,
Block B, Union Industrial Building, Singapore 2057

Library of Congress Cataloging-in-Publication Data

Parmar, Mahesh K.B.
    Survival analysis : a practical approach / Mahesh K.B. Parmar and
David Machin.
        p. cm.
    Includes bibliographical references and index.
    ISBN 0-471-93640-5 (hardcover)
    1. Survival analysis (Biometry)   I. Machin, David.   II. Title.
    R853.S7P37   1995
610'.72—dc20   95–32240
                                                              CIP

British Library Cataloguing in Publication Data

A catalogue record for this book is available from the British Library

ISBN 0 471 93640 5

Typeset in 10/12 pt Palatino by
Mathematical Composition Setters Ltd, Salisbury, Wiltshire, SP3 4UF

Printed and bound in Great Britain by
Bookcraft (Bath) Ltd, Midsomer Norton, Avon

This book is printed on acid-free paper responsibly manufactured from
sustainable forestation, for which at least two trees are planted for each one
used for paper production.

To
Ambaben B. Parmar
and
Annie Machin

Contents

Preface

Survival methods are used in many circumstances in medical and allied areas of research. Our objective here is to explain these methods in an accessible and non-technical way. We have assumed some familiarity with basic statistical ideas, but we have tried not to overwhelm the reader with details of statistical theory. Instead, we have tried to give a practical guide to the use of survival analysis techniques in a variety of situations by using numerous examples. A number of these arise from our own particular field of interest—cancer clinical trials—but the issues that arise in the analysis of such data are common to trials in general and to epidemiological studies.

There are many people whom we would like to thank: these include past and present members of the Medical Research Council Cancer Therapy Committee and its associated working parties, colleagues of the Human Reproduction Programme of the World Health Organization, the European School of Oncology and the Nordic School of Public Health.

Particular thanks go to Vicki Budd, Maria Dasseville, Vivien Ellen and Vicki Greaves for typing the many drafts of each chapter, to Philippa Lloyd for detailed comments on the final draft and Lesley Stewart for providing a general assessment of the book's accessibility. We also thank John Machin, Caroline Mallam and Andrea Bailey for their statistical computing, and John Machin again for keeping us organised.

Mahesh K. B. Parmar and David Machin

1 | Introduction and Review of Statistical Concepts

Summary

In this chapter we first introduce some examples of the use of survival methods in a selection of different areas. In the rest of the chapter we describe basic statistical ideas useful in survival analysis. These include the median survival, the Normal distribution and confidence intervals. We define the hazard ratio—the statistic commonly used to summarise the difference between two survival curves. We contrast the hazard ratio with the relative risk and odds ratio. We also introduce the idea of hypothesis testing; in particular, the test of the hypothesis that there is no difference between the survival of two groups, and we discuss the differences and similarities between hypothesis testing and the use of confidence intervals. We introduce the χ^2 (chi-squared) and likelihood ratio tests—two tests which are often used in survival analysis. We introduce these tests in their simplest form. We briefly discuss the difference between clinical and statistical significance. We end the chapter with a summary of some of the computing packages which can be used to analyse and manage survival data. This chapter is intended to serve largely as a reference chapter for readers to 'dip' into and read those sections on topics with which they are either unfamiliar or areas in which they require some clarification.

1.1 INTRODUCTION

There are many examples in medicine where a survival time measurement is appropriate. For example, such measurements may include the time a kidney graft remains functional, the time a patient with colorectal cancer survives once the tumour has been removed by surgery, the time a patient with osteoarthrosis is pain free following acupuncture treatment, the time a woman remains without a pregnancy whilst using a particular hormonal contraceptive and the time a pressure sore takes to heal. All these times are triggered by an initial event: a kidney graft, a surgical intervention, commencement of acupuncture therapy, first use of a contraceptive or identification of the pressure sore. These initial events are followed by a subsequent event: graft failure, death, return of pain, pregnancy or healing of the sore. The time between such events is known as the 'survival time'. The term *survival* is used because the first use of such techniques arose from the insurance industry, who were developing methods of costing insurance premiums. They needed to know the risk, or average survival time, associated with a particular type of client. This 'risk' was based on that of a large group of individuals with a particular age, sex and possibly other characteristics; the individual was then given the risk for his or her group for the calculation of insurance premiums.

There is one major difference between 'survival' data and other types of numeric continuous data: the time to the event occurring is not necessarily observed in all subjects. Thus in the above examples we may not observe for all subjects the events of graft failure (the graft remains functional indefinitely), death (the patient survives for a very long time), return of pain (the patient remains pain free thereafter), pregnancy (the woman never conceives) or healing of the sore (the sore does not heal), respectively. Such non-observed events are quite different from missing data items.

Example from the literature

One early example of the use of survival methods has been in the description of the subsequent survival experience and identification of risk factors associated with patients requiring heart transplants. Thus Table 1.1, adapted from Turnbull *et al.* (1974), reproduces some of the earliest heart transplant data published. The aim of a heart transplant programme is to restore the patient to the level of risk of his or her healthy contemporaries of the same age.

In a heart transplant programme, patients are assessed for transplant and then, if suitable, have to await a donor heart. One consequence of this wait is that patients may die before a suitable donor has been found (survival time X in Table 1.1). Thirty patients, of the 82 summarised in Table 1.1, did not actually receive a transplant. Of these, 27 died before a donor heart became available and three remained alive and were still waiting for a suitable transplant heart at 1 March 1973, for 118, 91 and 427 days, respectively. For those who receive a transplant their survival time is measured from the date of assessment of suitability and consists of their waiting time to transplant, Y, plus their survival time from their transplant until death, Z. Thus, for the third patient who received a transplant, the waiting time to a transplant is $Y = 50$ days and the survival post transplant is $Z = 624$ days. This patient, therefore, lived for $Y + Z = 50 + 624 = 674$ days from admission to the transplant programme.

The date of 1 March 1973 can be thought of as the 'census day', i.e. the day on

Table 1.1 Times to transplant and survival times for 82 patients selected for the Stanford Heart Transplantation Program (From Turnbull *et al.*, 1974. Reprinted with permission from *Journal of the American Statistical Association.* Copyright 1974 by the American Statistical Association. All rights reserved.)

30 patients not receiving a transplant by 1 March 1973		52 patients receiving a transplant by 1 March 1973					
X	State*	Y	Z	State	Y	Z	State
49	d	0	15	d	82	663	a
5	d	35	3	d	31	253	d
17	d	50	624	d	40	147	d
2	d	11	46	d	9	51	d
39	d	25	127	d	66	479	a
84	d	16	61	d	20	322	d
7	d	36	1350	d	77	442	a
0	d	27	312	d	2	65	d
35	d	19	24	d	26	419	a
36	d	17	10	d	32	362	a
1400	a	7	1024	d	13	64	d
5	d	11	39	d	56	228	d
34	d	2	730	d	2	65	d
15	d	82	136	d	9	264	a
11	d	24	1379	a	4	25	d
2	d	70	1	d	30	193	a
1	d	15	836	d	3	196	a
39	d	16	60	d	26	63	d
8	d	50	1140	a	4	12	d
101	d	22	1153	a	45	103	a
2	d	45	54	d	25	60	a
148	d	18	47	d	5	43	a
1	d	4	0	d			
68	d	1	43	d			
31	d	40	971	a			
1	d	57	868	a			
20	d	0	44	d			
118	a	1	780	a			
91	a	20	51	d			
427	a	35	710	a			

* a = alive, d = dead;
X = days to death or census date of 1 March 1973;
Y = days to transplant;
Z = days from transplant to death or census date.

which the currently available data on all patients recruited to the transplant programme were collected together and summarised. Typically, as in this example, by the census day some patients will have died whilst others remain alive. The survival times of those who are still alive are termed *censored survival times.* Censored survival times are described in section 2.1.

The probability of survival without transplant for patients identified as transplant candidates is shown in Figure 1.1. Details of how this probability is

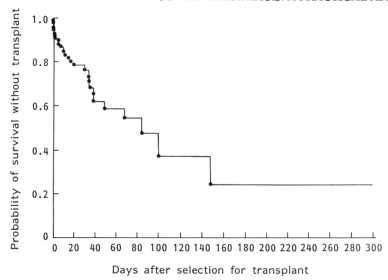

Figure 1.1 Probability of survival without transplant for transplant candidates. Estimated from all pre-transplant experience by the Kaplan–Meier method (From Turnbull *et al.*, 1974. Reprinted with permission from *Journal of the American Statistical Association*. Copyright 1974 by the American Statistical Association. All rights reserved.)

calculated using the Kaplan–Meier (product-limit) estimate, are given in section 2.4. By reading across from 0.5 on the vertical scale in Figure 1.1 and then vertically downwards at the point of intersection with the curve, we can say that approximately half (see section 2.6) of such patients will die within 80 days of being selected as suitable for transplant if no transplant becomes available for them. Thus the patients selected for the programme are clearly at very high risk of death. This is to be expected since patients are only chosen for transplant if they have a life-threatening heart condition.

Historically, much of survival analysis has been developed and applied in relation to cancer clinical trials in which the survival time is often measured from the date of randomisation or commencement of therapy until death. The seminal papers by Peto *et al.* (1976, 1977) published in the *British Journal of Cancer* describing the design, conduct and analysis of cancer trials provide a landmark in the development and use of survival methods.

Example from the literature

Peto *et al.* (1977) describe the survival experience of 102 patients with chronic granulocytic leukaemia (CGL) measured from the time of first treatment following diagnosis of their disease to the date of death. The 'life table' estimate of the percentage surviving is given in Figure 1.2 and shows that most patients have died by 300 weeks or approximately 6 years. The method of calculating such a survival curve is described in section 2.4. These patients with CGL were randomly allocated to receive either chemotherapy, in the form of busulphan, or radiotherapy treatment for their disease. The life table estimate of survival for each of the two

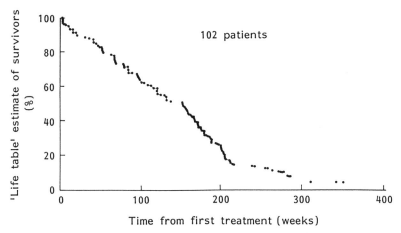

Figure 1.2 Life table for all patients in the Medical Research Council's first CGL trial. The numbers of patients alive and under observation at entry and annually thereafter were: 102, 84, 65, 50, 18, 11, 3 (reproduced from Peto *et al.*, 1977, by permission of The Macmillan Press Ltd)

treatment groups is shown in Figure 1.3 and suggests that the patients who received busulphan therapy lived, on average, longer than those who received radiotherapy. The method of making formal comparisons of two such survival curves with the logrank test is described in chapter 4, and the extension to more than two groups in chapter 5.

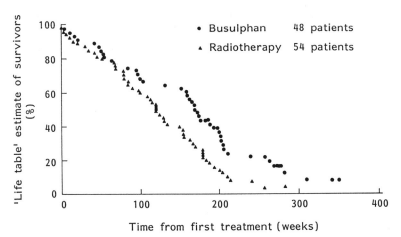

Figure 1.3 Life tables for the two separate treatment groups in the Medical Research Council's first CGL trial. The numbers of patients alive and under observation at entry and annually thereafter were: busulphan 48, 40, 33, 30, 13, 9, 3; and radiotherapy 54, 44, 32, 20, 3, 2, 0 (reproduced from Peto *et al.*, 1977, by permission of The Macmillan Press Ltd)

One field of application of survival studies has been in the development of methods of fertility regulation. In such applications alternative contraceptive methods either for the male or female partner are compared in prospective randomised trials. These trials usually compare the efficacy of different methods by observing how many women conceive in each group. A pregnancy is deemed a failure in this context. We discuss some special issues involved in contraceptive trials in chapter 10.

Example from the literature

It has been shown that gossypol, a plant extract, can lower the sperm count to render men temporarily sterile (azoospermic) and hence may be useful as a male contraceptive method. In a study of 46 men who had taken gossypol, and as a consequence had become azoospermic, their time to recovery of sperm function was recorded by Meng *et al.* (1988). This was measured from the date they stopped taking gossypol to recovery, defined as 'three successive semen samples with (summed) sperm concentration totalling at least 60×10^6/ml, provided none of the three counts was less than 15×10^6/ml'. The time to recovery was taken to be the time from the day they stopped taking gossypol to the date of first semen sample used in the above calculation. For those men who did not recover, their period of observation gives an incomplete or censored time to recovery at the date of the last semen sample.

The cumulative recovery rate to normal semen values for the 46 men is given in Figure 1.4 and suggests that approximately 70% of these men have recovered full sperm count in a little over 2 years from ceasing to use gossypol. Return to normal function is an important requirement of contraceptive methods if they are to be used to facilitate timing and spacing of pregnancies rather than just achieving permanent sterilisation.

Survival time methods have been used extensively in many medical fields, including cardiovascular disease (Packer *et al.*, 1991; Galloe *et al.*, 1993), chronic bronchitis (Multicenter Study Group, 1980), return of post-stroke function (Mayo *et al.*, 1991), and more recently AIDS (Aboulker and Swart, 1993). Other examples of the use of survival techniques are given throughout this book.

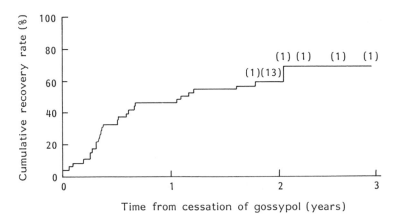

Figure 1.4 Cumulative recovery rate to threshold sperm function. Figures in parentheses indicate the follow-up time of the 18 men not yet recovered (reproduced from Meng *et al.*, 1988, by permission of Blackwell Science)

1.2 BASIC STATISTICAL IDEAS

The aim of nearly all studies, including those involving 'survival' data, is to extrapolate from observations made on a sample of individuals to the population as a whole. For example, in a trial of a new treatment for arthritis it is usual to assess the merits of the therapy on a sample of patients (preferably in a randomised controlled trial) and try to deduce from this trial whether the therapy is appropriate for general use in patients with arthritis. In many instances, it may be that the target population is more exactly specified, for example by patients with arthritis of a certain type, of a particular severity, or patients of a certain sex and age. Nevertheless, the aim remains the same: the inference from the results obtained from a sample to a (larger) population.

MEDIAN SURVIVAL

A commonly reported summary statistic in survival studies is the median survival time. The median survival time is defined as the value for which 50% of the individuals have longer survival times and 50% have shorter survival times. A more formal definition is given in section 2.6. The reason for reporting this value rather than the mean survival time is because the distributions of survival time data often tend to be skew, sometimes with a small number of long-term 'survivors'. The mean is defined in equation (1.1) below. For example, the distribution shown in Figure 1.5(a) of the delay between first symptom and formal diagnosis of cervical cancer in 131 women, ranging from 1 to 610 days, is not symmetric. The distribution is skewed to the right, in that the right-hand tail of the distribution is much longer than the left-hand tail. In this situation the mean is not a good summary of the 'average' survival time because it is unduly influenced by the extreme observations. The median delay to diagnosis for the women with cervical cancer was 135 days.

In this example, we have the duration of the delay in diagnosis for all 131 women. However, the approach used here for calculating the median should not be

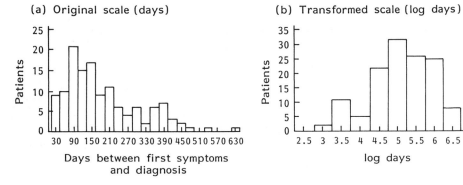

Figure 1.5 Distribution of the delay from first symptom to diagnosis of cervical cancer in 131 women. (a) Original scale (days). (b) Transformed scale (log days)

used if there are censored values amongst our observations. This will usually be the case with survival-type data. In this instance the method described in section 2.6 is appropriate.

THE NORMAL DISTRIBUTION

For many types of medical data the histogram of a continuous variable obtained from a single measurement on different subjects will have a characteristic 'bell-shaped' or Normal distribution. For some data which do not have such a distribution, a simple transformation of the variable may help. For example, if we calculate $x = \log t$ for each of the $n = 131$ women, where t is the delay from first symptom to diagnosis, then the distribution of x is given in Figure 1.5(b). This distribution is closer to the Normal distribution shape than that of Figure 1.5(a) and we can therefore calculate the arithmetic mean—more briefly the mean—of the x's by

$$\bar{x} = \Sigma x/n \tag{1.1}$$

to indicate the average value of the data illustrated in Figure 1.5(b). For these data, this gives $\bar{x} = 4.88$ log days.

Now that the distribution has an approximately Normal shape we can express the variability in values about the mean by the standard deviation (SD). This is given by

$$SD = \sqrt{[\Sigma(x - \bar{x})^2/(n - 1)]}. \tag{1.2}$$

For the women with delay to diagnosis of their cervical cancer, equation (1.2) gives $SD = 0.81$ log days. From this we can then calculate the standard error (SE) of the mean as

$$SE(\bar{x}) = SD/\sqrt{n}. \tag{1.3}$$

This gives $SE(\bar{x}) = 0.81/\sqrt{131} = 0.07$ log days.

CONFIDENCE INTERVALS

For any statistic, such as a mean, $\bar{x}$, it is useful to have an idea of the uncertainty in using this as an estimate of the underlying true mean, μ. This is done by constructing a (confidence) interval—a range of values around the estimate—which we can be confident includes the true underlying value. Such a confidence interval (CI) for the estimated mean extends evenly either side of the mean by a multiple of the standard error (SE) of the mean. Thus, for example, a 95% CI is the range of values from estimated mean $- (1.96 \times SE)$ to estimated mean $+ (1.96 \times SE)$, while a 99% CI is the range of values from estimated mean $- (2.5758 \times SE)$ to estimated mean $+ (2.5758 \times SE)$. In general a $100(1 - \alpha)\%$ CI, for the estimated mean, $\bar{x}$, is given by

$$\bar{x} - z_{1-\alpha/2} \times SE(\bar{x}) \quad \text{to} \quad \bar{x} + z_{1-\alpha/2} \times SE(\bar{x}). \tag{1.4}$$

Here $z_{1-\alpha/2}$ and $-z_{1-\alpha/2}$ are the upper and lower $1 - \alpha/2$ points of the standard Normal distribution of Figure 1.6, respectively.

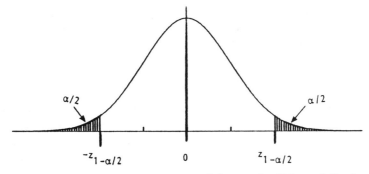

Figure 1.6 Upper and lower $\alpha/2$ points of the standard Normal distribution

Example

For the data of Figure 1.5b suppose we require a 95% CI for log μ, the log of the true underlying mean. Then $\alpha = 0.05$ and $1 - \alpha/2 = 0.975$. From Table T1 locating the cell 0.0500 or in Table T2 using two-sided $\alpha = 0.0500$, we obtain $z_{0.975} = 1.96$. Substituting $\bar{x} = 4.88$, SE $= 0.07$ and $z_{0.975} = 1.96$ in equation (1.4) gives a 95% CI for log μ as 4.7428 to 5.017 log days. To obtain a 95% CI for μ, as opposed to log μ, we antilog the lower and upper values of our CI to obtain $\exp(4.7428) = 115$ and $\exp(5.017) = 151$ days, respectively.

As already indicated, we can increase the probability of including the true mean in the CI to, say, 99% by multiplying the SE in equation (1.4) by 2.5758 from Table T2 in place of 1.96. This 99% CI will be wider, and thus represent greater uncertainty, than the corresponding 95% interval. Similarly we could reduce the probability to 90% by multiplying the SE by 1.6449 from Table T2, which, in turn, reduces the width of the interval. For no other reason than convention, it is common to report 95% CIs.

The expressions for the summary statistics and their SEs are different for different situations and some of these are listed in Table 1.2. Thus if a CI is required for the proportion of responses to a particular therapy, then we require to estimate this

Table 1.2 Some summary statistics and their standard errors (SE)

Statistic	Population value	Estimate	Standard error (SE)
Mean	μ	$\bar{x} = \Sigma\, x/n$	$SD/\sqrt{n}$
Difference between two means	$\delta = \mu_A - \mu_B$	$d = \bar{x}_A - \bar{x}_B$	$\sqrt{\left(\dfrac{SD_A^2}{n_A} + \dfrac{SD_B^2}{n_B} \right)}$
Proportion	π	$p = r/n$	$\sqrt{\left[\dfrac{p(1-p)}{n} \right]}$
Difference between two proportions	$\delta = \pi_A - \pi_B$	$d = p_A - p_B$	$\sqrt{\left[\dfrac{p_A(1-p_A)}{n_A} + \dfrac{p_B(1-p_B)}{n_B} \right]}$

proportion by $p = r/n$, where r is the number of responses in n patients, and the $SE = \sqrt{[p(1-p)/n]}$ as indicated in Table 1.2. These are then substituted in equation (1.4) in place of $\bar{x}$ and $SE(\bar{x})$, respectively, to obtain a CI. Further details of the calculation and use of CIs are given by Gardner and Altman (1989).

A particularly important application of the use of estimation is to make a statement about relative treatment efficacy in a randomised clinical trial of, say, a new therapy compared to a standard or control treatment for a particular condition. The CI provides a range of values in which the true effect is likely to lie. That is, there is a small chance that this range will not contain the true effect. With a 95% CI there is a 5% chance that the true effect does not lie within it, while with a 99% CI there is only a 1% chance.

Example from the literature

The results of a clinical trial conducted by Familiari *et al.* (1981) comparing two drugs for the treatment of peptic ulcers are summarised in Table 1.3. Of 61 patients recruited 30 received Pirenzepine (P) and 31 Trithiozine (T) and the proportions not healed are, respectively, 23% and 42%.

Table 1.3 Percentage of peptic ulcers healed by treatment group (after Familiari *et al.*, 1981)

Drug	Not healed	Healed	Total	Percentage not healed
Pirenzepine (P)	7 (a)	23 (c)	30(c + a)	23.33
Trithiozine (T)	13 (b)	18 (d)	31(d + b)	41.94
Total	20 (r)	41 (s)	61 (N)	

In an obvious notation $n_p = 30$, $p_p = a/(c + a) = 0.2333$, $n_T = 31$ and $p_T = b/(d + b) = 0.4194$. The observed difference between treatments is $d = p_T - p_P = 0.4194 - 0.2333 = 0.1861$. The corresponding SE of d is given in Table 1.2 by

$$SE(d) = \sqrt{\left[\frac{p_T(1 - p_T)}{n_T} + \frac{p_P(1 - p_P)}{n_p}\right]}$$

$$= 0.1175.$$

From equation (1.6) the 95% CI around the difference in proportions is -0.0442 to 0.4164 or -4% to $+42\%$. Thus, although there are more unhealed patients with Trithiozine, the 95% CI does not exclude the possibility that the true difference between treatments may be zero.

1.3   THE HAZARD RATIO

The hazard ratio (HR) has been specifically developed for survival data, and is used as a measure of the relative survival experience of two groups. It is described in detail in chapter 4. In brief, if the observed number of deaths in group A is O_A and the corresponding expected number of deaths (under the hypothesis of no survival difference between the groups under study) is E_A then the ratio O_A/E_A is the relative death rate or relative hazard in group A. Similarly O_B/E_B is the relative death rate or relative hazard in group B. The HR is then defined as

$$HR = \frac{O_A/E_A}{O_B/E_B}. \qquad (1.5)$$

The HR is the ratio of the relative hazards in the two groups. It is important to note that for the HR the 'expected' deaths in both groups are calculated using the logrank method described in chapter 4. This method allows for the censoring which occurs in nearly all survival data. The HR gives an estimate of the overall difference between the survival curves as discussed in section 4.3. If there is no difference between two groups the value of $HR = 1$, and this can be tested by means of the logrank test of section 4.2.

However, summarising the difference between two survival curves into one statistic can also have its problems. One particularly important consideration for its use is that the ratio of the relative hazards in the two groups should not vary greatly over time. Section 6.1 describes a graphical approach to assessing this.

RELATIVE RISK

The term *relative risk* (RR) has been defined for use in prospective epidemiological or cohort studies, in which groups of subjects with different exposures to a potential hazard are followed to see whether or not an event of interest occurs. Thus Table 1.4 represents the notation for a prospective study in which two groups of industrial workers are likely to be exposed to different types of asbestos. They are then followed in time to see if they do or do not develop mesothelioma (the event under study). We assume here that all these workers are examined for evidence of the disease at, say, 15 years following their first exposure, and only presence or absence of the disease noted at that time.

A total of N subjects have been followed, $(c + a)$ who were exposed to Type I asbestos and $(d + b)$ exposed to Type II asbestos. The proportions of subjects in which mesothelioma subsequently develops, as recorded 15 years later, are $a/(c + a)$

Table 1.4 General representation of the results of a prospective epidemiological study in the form of a 2×2 table

Asbestos	Mesothelioma diagnosed		Total
	Yes	No	
Type I	a	c	(c + a)
Type II	b	d	(d + b)
Total	r	s	N

and $b/(d+b)$ for Types I and II asbestos respectively. The RR is the ratio of these two proportions and is a measure of increased (or decreased) risk in one group when compared with the other. Thus

$$RR = \frac{a/(c+a)}{b/(d+b)}$$

$$= \frac{a(d+b)}{b(c+a)}. \qquad (1.6)$$

If there is no difference between the two exposure groups, i.e. the Type of asbestos exposure does not influence the proportion of individuals subsequently developing mesothelioma, the expected value of the RR = 1.

Example

To illustrate the calculation of a RR we use the data of Table 1.3, although this summarises a clinical trial rather than an epidemiological investigation. These data give, from equation (1.6), RR = $(7 \times 31)/(13 \times 30) = 0.5564$ or approximately 0.6. This suggests that those patients receiving Pirenzepine are at approximately half the risk of their ulcers not healing as those who receive Trithiozine.

ODDS RATIO

Using the same layout as in Table 1.4 we can define the odds of developing to not developing mesothelioma with Type I asbestos as $a:c$ and similarly as $b:d$ for Type II asbestos. The odds ratio (OR) is defined as:

$$OR = \frac{a/c}{b/d} = \frac{ad}{bc}. \qquad (1.7)$$

If there is no difference in the odds of developing mesothelioma in the two asbestos groups then the expected value of OR = 1.

Example

In the example of Table 1.3 we have a = 7, b = 13, c = 23 and d = 18. Hence a/c is 7/23 and b/d is 13/18, giving an OR = $(7 \times 18)/(13 \times 23) = 0.42$.

In this example, an OR < 1 indicates more unhealed ulcers with Trithiozine as we had concluded when we calculated the RR = 0.5. The values of the RR and OR are quite similar here and we return to this below.

RELATIONSHIP BETWEEN THE HR, RR AND OR

If we return to Table 1.4 and consider situations when the event is rare, i.e. relatively few individuals will get mesothelioma from a large number of workers exposed to asbestos, then the number a will be small compared with the number c. In this case $a/(c+a)$ will be approximately equal to a/c. Similarly $b/(d+b)$ will be approximately equal to b/d. As a consequence, in this situation, equation (1.5) for the RR is approximately

$$RR \simeq \frac{a/c}{b/d} = \frac{ad}{bc}. \tag{1.8}$$

Thus both the OR and RR can be calculated for the situation in the example of Table 1.3 and, in fact in this case, they are not numerically too dissimilar.

However, in a retrospective case–control study, only the OR can be estimated. This is because, if the numerical procedure of equation (1.6) is used to calculate the RR directly in a case–control study, the result obtained depends on the proportion of cases to controls selected by the design. For example, if one doubles the number of controls the OR remains the same since we double both the numerator and denominator in equation (1.7), but the value obtained for the RR will be different. Nevertheless, in situations in which the event is rare, the OR may provide an estimate of the corresponding RR.

We have now seen that the OR and RR can be numerically similar, and that the OR can provide an estimate of the RR when the event rates are small. There is also a link between the HR and RR and in special situations the HR can be the same as the RR. This is best shown by an example.

Example

Suppose that Familiari *et al.* (1981) had recorded the time to ulcer healing in their patients, but then had decided to ignore this information and just report the responses to treatment at a fixed time (say) 3 months from start of therapy. In this case, those patients with healed ulcers within 3 months will be included as healed in Table 1.3 but those which heal after this time will not be counted.

If we were to analyse these data using standard methods for a 2×2 table then under the (null) hypothesis of no difference in outcome in the two groups, the expected proportion of unhealed ulcers in the two groups will be estimated, using the same notation as before, by $(a+b)/N = r/N$. Of these, we would expect $E_P = (c+a) \times (r/N) = r(c+a)/N$ to occur in those patients treated with Pirenzepine and $E_T = (d+b) \times (r/N) = r(d+b)/N$ to occur in those treated with Trithiozine. Now the actual numbers of unhealed ulcers in groups P and T are $O_P = a$ and $O_T = b$, respectively. Hence if we were then to use equation (1.5) we would have

$$HR = \frac{O_P/E_P}{O_T/E_T} = \frac{a/[r(c+a)/N]}{b/[r(d+b/N]}$$

$$= \frac{a/(c+a)}{b/(d+b)} = \frac{a(d+b)}{b(c+a)}.$$

Reference to equation (1.6) shows that this is just the expression for the RR. Thus, when there is no censoring (see section 2.1) and when the actual time an event occurs is not considered important, and is not therefore used, the HR and RR are equivalent.

As mentioned above, there is some confusion in the appropriate use of the RR and OR and this extends to the use of the HR. The HR is specifically defined for survival studies in which the time between two critical events is recorded. In these circumstances, the HR is the estimate which should always be used and reported.

Despite this many researchers still refer to the 'HR' as the 'RR'. This is poor practice and we prefer to use the terminology of HR for survival studies and reserve the term RR for situations in which both censoring, and the time at which the critical event occurs, are not relevant.

1.4   SIGNIFICANCE TESTS

A central feature of statistical analysis is the test of the null hypothesis of 'no difference'. For example, in a clinical trial of a new treatment versus a standard treatment the null hypothesis that is to be tested is that there is no difference between the new and standard treatments in their efficacy.

To test the null hypothesis, often denoted by H_0, we compare the group of patients receiving the new treatment with the group receiving the standard, with the goal of rejecting the null hypothesis in favour of an alternative hypothesis, should a difference in efficacy be observed. Such an alternative hypothesis, often denoted H_A, is that there is a real difference between the new and the standard therapies in their efficacy.

The z-test, which is used as the significance test of the null hypothesis, takes the form

$$z = \frac{(\text{Observed difference}) - (\text{difference anticipated by the null hypothesis})}{\text{SE(Observed difference)}}. \quad (1.9)$$

In many circumstances, the estimate of the effect anticipated by the null hypothesis is zero, so that equation (1.9) becomes, in such cases,

$$z = \frac{(\text{Observed difference})}{\text{SE(Observed difference)}} \quad (1.10)$$

Once the test statistic z is calculated, then its value is referred to Table T1 of the Normal distribution to obtain the p-value.

The resulting p-value is defined as the answer to the question: what is the probability that we would have observed the difference, *or a more extreme difference*, if the null hypothesis was true?

Example

In the context of the trial of two treatments for peptic ulcers by Familiari *et al.* (1981) the null hypothesis is that both Pirenzipine and Trithiozine are equally effective in healing peptic ulcers. The observed difference between the treatments is expressed in terms of $d = 0.1861$. The corresponding null hypothesis of no treatment difference is stated as δ, the true difference, equals zero.

Thus, use of equation (1.10) with the Observed difference $d = 0.1861$ and the SE(Observed difference) = SE(d) = 0.1175, gives $z = 0.1861/0.1175 = 1.58$. Reference to Table T1, with $z = 1.58$, gives a total area in the tails of the distribution, by combining that to the left of $z = -1.58$ with that to the right of $z = +1.58$, of 0.1141. This area is termed the p-value.

If the p-value is small, say <0.001, then we may conclude that the null hypothesis is unlikely to be true. On the other hand, if the p-value is large, say >0.5, we would be reluctant to conclude that it is not true.

However, somewhere between these two clear possibilities there is likely to be a grey area in which it is hard to decide. For this reason, it has become something of a convention to report a 'statistically significant' result if the p-value <0.05, and a 'highly statistically significant' result if the p-value <0.01. However, the exact value of the p-value obtained in these circumstances should always be quoted. It is a somewhat unfortunate convention to use 'not statistically significant' if the p-value >0.05. It is particularly important in this latter situation to quote the exact p-value, the value of the estimate of the difference (OR, RR or HR) and the corresponding CI.

Example

In the case of the p-value = 0.1141 obtained from the significance test from the data on peptic ulcers, then this is clearly >0.05. From this we may conclude that there is no statistically significant difference between the healing rates of the two drugs. This does not imply, as we have already indicated, that the treatments are necessarily equal in efficacy, only that we cannot say that there is sufficient evidence of a difference from the data provided by this trial.

SIGNIFICANCE TESTS AND CONFIDENCE INTERVALS

As we have discussed in the context of a randomised trial, the estimate of the difference between the treatments obtained with the trial data is the best estimate of the true or population value. Further the CI provides a range of values, in particular plausible minimum and maximum values in which the effect is likely to lie. A hypothesis test does not tell us about the actual size of the effect, only whether it is likely to be different from zero.

Although the two approaches of CIs and significance tests do apparently address different questions, there is a close relationship between them. For example, whenever the 95% CI for the estimate excludes the value zero, i.e. the CI lies either entirely above or entirely below zero, then the corresponding hypothesis test will usually yield a p-value <0.05. Similarly, if the 99% CI for the estimate excludes zero, then the p-value <0.01.

In succeeding chapters, we may if the context is very clear replace 'p-value = 0.023' by the shortened form 'p = 0.023'.

1.5   CLINICAL AND STATISTICAL SIGNIFICANCE

It is important to distinguish between a 'clinically significant' result and a 'statistically significant' result. The former is an effect, which if established, is likely to make a real (clinical) impact. For example, if the difference in efficacy between two treatments, as established by a randomised clinical trial, is substantial then the better of the two treatments if given to all future patients will have clinical impact and is therefore 'clinically significant'. In certain circumstances, even small differences that are firmly established may have clinical impact. For example, the impact of aspirin in reducing the risk of second attacks in patients who have suffered a myocardial infarction is not dramatic, but the modest benefit gained through its use has been shown to save many lives annually since the disease is common. Hence, although the effect is small, the result is of considerable 'clinical significance'.

In contrast, a statistically significant result does not automatically imply a clinically important consequence of that result. For example, suppose we demonstrate that a new therapy provides a small but statistically significant improvement in survival over the standard therapy: however, the new therapy is so toxic, difficult and costly that the small improvement in survival is not sufficient to make it clinically worthwhile to use the new therapy in patients. Consequently, the trial has produced a statistically significant result of little clinical significance.

It is also necessary to appreciate that one should not dismiss a result that is 'not statistically significant' as therefore not clinically important—for example, a study may be too small to reliably detect and measure important differences between two treatments. In this situation the study may provide an estimate of the difference which, had it been reliably shown and measured, would have been of clinical importance. In such circumstances it may be that the study should be repeated, perhaps in a larger group of patients. We discuss the choice of sample sizes for survival studies in chapter 10.

We now introduce two additional methods for performing significance tests which form the basis of many of the tests used in the remainder of the book.

1.6   THE χ^2 TEST

We have seen earlier, when discussing the relation between the HR, OR and RR, that the analysis of data from a randomised trial comparing two groups can be expressed in terms of observed (O) and expected (E) values. In the notation of Table 1.3, we have observed, for the four cells of the table, $O_1 = a$, $O_2 = b$, $O_3 = c$ and $O_4 = d$. The corresponding expected values, calculated on the assumption of the null hypothesis of no difference, are $E_1 = r(c + a)/N$, $E_2 = r(d + b)/N$, $E_3 = s(c + a)/N$ and $E_4 = s(d + b)/N$. These values are then substituted into

$$\chi^2 = \Sigma (O - E)^2/E \tag{1.11}$$

where the summation is over the four cells of Table 1.3. Such a table is often termed a (2×2) contingency table with $R = 2$ rows and $C = 2$ columns. We use a similar equation to (1.11) when describing the logrank test in chapter 4.

Example

Using the data of Familiari et al. (1981), $O_1 = 7$, $O_2 = 13$, $O_3 = 23$ and $O_4 = 18$. The corresponding expected values are $E_1 = 9.8361$, $E_2 = 10.1639$, $E_3 = 20.1639$ and $E_4 = 20.8361$. This gives

$$\chi^2 = \frac{(7 - 9.8361)^2}{9.8361} + \frac{(13 - 10.1639)^2}{10.1639} + \frac{(23 - 20.1639)^2}{20.1639} + \frac{(18 - 20.8361)^2}{20.8361} = 2.3941.$$

The value $\chi^2 = 2.39$ is then referred to Table T3 of the χ^2 distribution with degrees of freedom (df) equal to one. This gives the p-value ≈ 0.15. An exact value can be obtained in this case, since df = 1, by referring $z = \sqrt{(\chi^2)} = 1.5473$ to Table T1. Hence the p-value = 0.1141. We note that 1.5473 is close to $z = 1.58$ obtained from the use of equation (1.10). In fact, the two approaches are algebraically similar.

The basic concept of a χ^2 test, in the form of equation (1.11), can be extended to a general $R \times C$ contingency table. The number of degrees of freedom is now df = $(R - 1)(C - 1)$. The χ^2 test statistic obtained from the calculation corresponding to the $R \times C$ table is referred to Table T3 with the appropriate df.

1.7   THE LIKELIHOOD RATIO TEST

In some situations, an alternative approach to testing hypotheses is required. One such method is termed the likelihood ratio (LR) test. Such a test compares the probability or likelihood of the data under one hypothesis with the likelihood under an alternative hypothesis. To illustrate this procedure it is first necessary to define the likelihood of the data.

Suppose we are estimating the probability of response to treatment in a group of n patients with a particular disease and the true or population value for this probability is π. Then an individual patient will respond with probability π and fail to respond with probability $(1 - \pi)$. π must take a value between 0, the value when no patients ever respond, and 1, in which case all respond.

If, in our study, r of these patients respond and $(n - r)$ do not respond, then the probability of this outcome is proportional to

$$l = \pi^r (1 - \pi)^{(n-r)}. \tag{1.12}$$

Here l is termed the likelihood. If we then calculate L = log l then this is termed the log likelihood and we have

$$L = \log l = r \log \pi + (n - r) \log (1 - \pi). \tag{1.13}$$

It turns out that if we estimate π by p = r/n then this corresponds to the value for π which maximises the value of l in equation (1.12) or, equivalently, the maximum possible value of L in equation (1.13). We therefore state that p = r/n is the maximum likelihood estimate (mle) of π.

To obtain this estimate in a formal way, it is necessary to differentiate equation (1.13) with respect to π and equate the result to zero. The solution of this equation gives the estimate for π as r/n.

The LR test calculates the likelihood under two different hypotheses and compares these. For convenience, we term these the likelihood under the null hypothesis, l_0, and the likelihood under the alternative hypothesis, l_A. The likelihood ratio test is then

$$LR = -2\log(l_0/l_A) = -2(L_0 - L_A).\qquad(1.14)$$

A large value of LR would indicate that the assumption of equal treatment efficacy is unlikely to be consistent with the data. If the null hypothesis were true we would expect a small value of the LR. In fact, it can be shown that the LR in equation (1.14) is approximately distributed as a χ^2 variable with the appropriate df.

The df corresponds to the difference between the number of parameters estimated under the alternative hypothesis, m_A, minus the number of parameters estimated under the null hypothesis, m_0, that is $df = m_A - m_0$. The value of the LR statistic is then referred to the χ^2 distribution, using the appropriate row in Table T3 for the df, to give the p-value.

Example

For the trial of Familiari *et al.* (1981) the null hypothesis is that $OR = 1$ or $\pi_P = \pi_T = \pi_0$. In this case we have one parameter π_0 which is estimated, using the notation of Table 1.3, by $r/N = 20/61$. Therefore, under the null hypothesis, equation (1.13) becomes

$$L_0 = r\log \pi_0 + (N - r) \log(1 - \pi_0)$$
$$= 20\log(20/61) + 41\log(41/61) = -38.5922.$$

In contrast, under the alternative hypothesis the two treatments differ and we estimate both parameters, π_P and π_T, separately by 7/30 and 13/31, respectively. In this case L_A, the log likelihood corresponding to equation (1.13), becomes the sum of L_P and L_T. That is,

$$L_A = L_P + L_T$$
$$= 7\log(7/30) + 23\log(23/30) + 13\log(13/31) + 18\log(18/31) = -37.3807.$$

Substituting these values for L_0 and L_A into equation (1.14) gives $LR = -2(-38.5922 + 37.3807) = 2.4230$. Reference to Table T3 with $df = 1$ gives a p-value >0.1 for this observed LR. To obtain a more precise figure for the p-value, in the case of $df = 1$ only, we calculate $z = \sqrt{(LR)} = 1.5566 = 1.56$ and refer this to Table T1 to obtain a p-value = 0.1188.

Finally we note that $z = 1.56$ is close to the $z = 1.58$ we obtained earlier using equation (1.10). These will often be close, although the two approaches are not algebraically equivalent. In our example, both the z and the LR tests yield much the same conclusion.

The advantage of the LR test of equation (1.14), over the z test of equation (1.9), is that the method extends to comparisons of more than two groups. For example, if we were comparing three treatments, then we would estimate three parameters, π_1, π_2 and π_3, under the alternative hypothesis and one parameter, π_0, under the null hypothesis. In this case $df = m_A - m_0 = 3 - 1 = 2$ and to obtain a p-value $= 0.05$, for example, in Table T3 we require a value of $\chi^2 = 5.99$ as opposed to $\chi^2 = 3.84$ when $df = 1$.

The maximum likelihood estimates of the parameters of both the exponential and Weibull distributions of survival are given in chapter 3 and further discussion of the LR statistic is given in chapter 6.

1.8   STATISTICAL COMPUTING

Many statistical packages now include procedures that enable the techniques described in this book to be implemented. Unfortunately that much of what we describe in this book cannot be implemented without good statistical package support. A comprehensive review of three packages used extensively for survival analysis—BMDP, SAS and SPSS—is given by Collett (1994). Other packages that have survival analysis facilities include EGRET, STATA and SYSTAT. The choice of package for use in your analysis may depend on the type of computer that you have available, although PC versions of statistical packages are becoming increasingly available and flexible.

It is important too that the data you collect can interface with these statistical packages. In many situations, particularly in clinical trials and longitudinal follow-up studies in epidemiology, the data do not come neatly packaged in a rectangular array, free of missing values and with complete information on the relevant endpoints for all subjects. Typically such studies have ragged data files of variable length for each subject. For example, those patients that die early following diagnosis of their disease will have a correspondingly short data file, while those that survive will have a long period of observation and a data file which continues to expand with time. Such ragged data files usually have to be converted to a flat file for transport to a statistical package.

In studies in which times between successive events are important, data base facilities must be readily available to calculate survival times by subtraction of two dates. Thus, in a patient recruited to a clinical trial with a fatal disease, the date of entry (DOE) to a trial therapy (first event) may be recorded, the patient is then followed up (FU) at successive clinical visits, each of which will have a date, DFU (1), DFU (2), ..., until his eventual death (DOD), which is the second (critical) event. The data base package must then have the facility to calculate the survival time in days by $t = DOD - DOE$. For those patients who have not died at the time of analysis (these create censored observations, see section 2.1) it is necessary to identify the last follow-up visit for each patient and determine that date. This is then used to calculate the (censored) survival time by $T^+ = DFU (Last) - DOE$. The facility to do such calculations easily is not routinely provided in most data base packages.

One set of data management facilities especially designed for longitudinal studies involving patient follow-up is available through COMPACT (COMPACT Steering Committee, 1991).

1.9 BIBLIOGRAPHY

As already indicated, important papers describing survival time applications in clinical trials are those by Peto *et al.* (1976, 1977). These papers describe not only appropriate statistical methodology but also many practical aspects relevant to the conduct of clinical trials. The book by Pocock (1983) provides a comprehensive description of clinical trial methodology. There are several explanatory papers presenting statistical methods for survival studies, including a description of the Cox regression model, and these include Christensen (1987) and Tibsharani (1982).

Mantel and Haenszel (1959) first described the product-limit estimator of the survival curve (chapter 2). The paper by Cox (1972) introducing the proportional hazards model (chapter 6), has led to a revolution in the analysis of survival data. There are several texts which describe survival analysis techniques but more from a technical perspective and they include, in approximate order of mathematical complexity, Marubini and Valsecchi (1995), Lee (1992), Gross and Clark (1975), Collett (1994), Cox and Oakes (1984) and Kabfleisch and Prentice (1980). These papers and books are written, however, for a more mathematical audience and may be heavy going for the general reader.

Basic statistical texts include Campbell and Machin (1993), Bland (1987) and Altman (1991) and these are ordered here in terms of their relative complexity and detail. The first is for beginners, the last for medical researchers. A full description of the use and calculation of CIs, including a computer package for implementation, is given by Gardner and Altman (1989).

Tables for the calculation of the appropriate size of a study required (chapter 10) when survival time endpoints are relevant are given by Machin and Campbell (1987). Advanced texts on epidemiological methods, and which also refer to survival applications, are Clayton and Hills (1993) and Breslow and Day (1980, 1987).

2 | Survival Curves

Summary

In this chapter we describe the basic methods that can be used to describe and analyse survival data involving censored observations. In particular, we present the method of calculating the Kaplan–Meier survival curve and associated confidence intervals. We also describe the calculation of the median survival time and introduce the use of the hazard rate.

2.1 SURVIVAL TIME DATA

In a clinical trial or medical investigation, patients are usually entered into the study over a period of time and then followed beyond the treatment or intervention period and assessed for the endpoint of interest some time later. However, as noted in chapter 1, this endpoint may not always be observed for all patients. For example, in a randomised trial of two radiotherapy doses in the treatment of cancer of the brain conducted by the Medical Research Council Brain Tumour Working Party (Bleehen *et al.*, 1991), 443 eligible patients were entered between April 1983 and September 1988. Thus recruitment to the trial lasted for almost 5½ years. The focus in this trial was to establish the influence of treatment on the length of patient survival from commencement of treatment until death. This event, i.e. the 'death', was considered the 'principal endpoint' of the trial. An analysis of this trial was performed early in 1990, at which time patients had differing times in the trial depending on their actual date of recruitment and hence the start of therapy. A total of 21 of the 443 patients were still alive at this analysis date. Although this is generally a fatal disease, for the analysis and reporting of the trial results it was unrealistic to wait until these 21 patients had died as some patients can live for a long time following diagnosis.

However, each of the 21 patients alive at the time of analysis had individual survival times from commencement of treatment. These ranged from 14 months in one patient who was entered rather late in the recruitment period, to 60 months (5 years) for one patient entered in the early stages of the trial. Thus for the patient who has survived 60 months, and is still alive, all we know is his total survival time from start of treatment to death will exceed 60 months. We denote this as 60+ months. If the analysis had been delayed until all the patients had died, the investigators may have had to wait for some considerable time, particularly if the patient with a survival time of 14+ months lived also for more than 5 years. Clearly, to wait for such an event would not have been advisable as it is important to report the conclusions from a study as soon as it is practically possible.

Further, some patients who have 'not yet died' may have actually 'left' the study, perhaps moving to a different locality or country. In such cases the investigators may never observe an 'event' for them. These patients are often termed 'lost to follow-up'.

Survival time is measured from one event, here start of treatment, to a subsequent event, here patient death. Patients for whom we have not observed the event of interest are said to provide 'censored' data. All we know about these patients is that they have survived a certain length of time. The reasons for this censoring are either that the patient has not yet died or that the patient has been lost to follow-up.

For the heart transplant patients of chapter 1, the 'survival' times may be the time from the date of diagnosis to the date a donor heart becomes available or, for

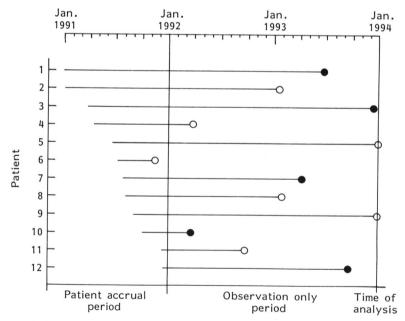

Figure 2.1 Patients entering a prospective clinical study at different times with the known (•) and censored (o) survival times indicated

those who receive a transplant, the time from surgery until rejection of the donor heart.

The flow of patients recruited to a typical prospective clinical study involving patient accrual and observation over time is illustrated in Figure 2.1. The study has a recruitment and observation phase, an observation only phase, and an analysis time.

In this trial, recruitment has been over a period of 1 year, further observations made for the next 2 years and the definitive analysis undertaken 3 years from the start of the trial. The maximum possible (observable) survival time for the two patients entered in early January 1991 is 3 years, whilst for the one recruited in late December 1991 it is only 2 years.

Figure 2.1 shows that five patients died and two were still alive at the end of the study. Five patients were lost from observation before the time of analysis and two were known to be alive and still under observation at the time of analysis. We often do not need to distinguish between the five patients lost to follow-up and for whom we could obtain no further information, and the two known to be alive at the date of analysis but who could be observed beyond the analysis date if necessary. We thus have five firm survival times and seven censored times. The patient recruitment dates, time at entry and time at death measured in days from 1 January 1991, and total survival time, are as shown in Table 2.1. The plus sign (+) denotes a censored survival time.

In most circumstances the different starting times of the patients are not relevant to the analysis of survival data, and neither is it necessary for the details in the third and fourth columns of the table to be recorded. However, it is necessary to order (or rank) the patient observations by the duration of the individual 'survival' times and Figure 2.2 shows the data of Figure 2.1 rearranged in rank order.

Table 2.1 Survival times for patients shown in Figure 2.1

Patient	Date of entry	Time at entry (days)	Time at death or censoring (days)	Dead (D) or censored (C)	Survival time (days)
1	01.01.91	0	910	D	910
2	01.01.91	0	752	C	752 +
3	26.03.91	86	1092	D	1006
4	26.04.91	116	452	C	336 +
5	23.06.91	175	1098	C	923 +
6	09.07.91	190	308	C	118 +
7	22.07.91	203	817	D	614
8	02.08.91	214	763	C	549 +
9	01.09.91	244	1098	C	854 +
10	07.10.91	280	432	D	152
11	14.12.91	348	645	C	297 +
12	26.12.91	360	1001	D	641

+, censored observation

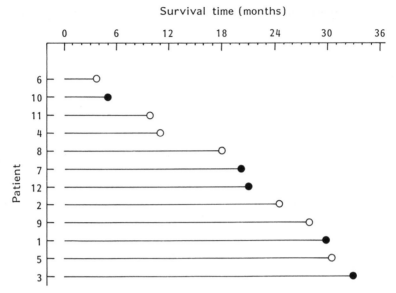

Figure 2.2   The data of Figure 2.1 ordered by length of observed survival time with (•) representing a known survival time and (o) a censored survival time

Example from the literature

McIllmurray and Turkie (1987) report the ordered survival times of 24 patients with Dukes' C colorectal cancer as 3+, 6, 6, 6, 6, 8, 8, 12, 12, 12+, 15+, 16+, 18+, 18+, 20, 22+, 24, 28+, 28+, 28+, 30, 30+, 33+ and 42 months.

These data, in the ordered format of Figure 2.2, are illustrated in Figure 2.3.

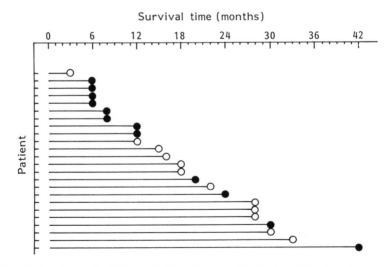

Figure 2.3   Ordered survival time of 24 patients with Dukes' C colorectal cancer (From McIllmurray and Turkie, 1987. Reproduced by permission of *Br. Med. J.* 294: 1260 and 295: 475. (Published by BMJ Publishing Group))

These same data are detailed again in Table 2.2. We will show in chapter 10 that, for assessing studies which involve patient follow-up, it is the number of critical events observed which is more important for statistical power considerations, rather than the number of patients actually recruited. Thus, all other considerations being equal, the study by McIllmurray and Turkie (1987) lacks statistical power, as only 12 patients (50%) had died at the time of analysis and reporting, while the remaining 12 (50%) were still alive. However, even if the authors had awaited the deaths of these patients the study would still have involved relatively few events (deaths). This contrasts with the Medical Research Council Brain Tumour Working Party trial in which 422 deaths (95% of the possible events) had occurred at the time of analysis.

The survival times of the patients with Dukes' C colorectal cancer in the McIllmurray and Turkie study are given to the nearest month resulting in, for example, four patients having the same recorded survival time of 6 months. Such observations are termed *tied*. It is usually better to avoid tied observations, if possible, and here if survival times had been reported in days then these four patients would be more likely to have different survival times, each of approximately 6 months. This would have allowed these four survival times to be placed in rank order, leading to the possibility of a more sensitive analysis.

Another feature of these data are the three patients with survival times of 12 months. Two of these patients have died at this time and the third is still alive. In ranking survival times it is a convention to give the censored observations in such a situation the higher rank. The assumption here is that the censored individual at, say, 12 months is likely to live longer than the patient who has died at 12 months even though the observation periods (as far as the study is concerned) are the same for these two individuals. The three survival times would thus be recorded as 12, 12 and 12+, having ranks 8, 9 and 10, respectively.

2.2   NOTATION

It is convenient to denote the observed survival time by (lower case) t for those observations in which the critical (second) event has occurred. However, as already indicated, there are often censored survival times in such studies which correspond to individuals in which the second event has not occurred. We denote their censored survival times by (capital) T^+. We might have used t^+ for this but, for expository purposes only, we use T^+ to give added emphasis to the fact that they are censored observations. Observed individual survival times are distinguished by using a subscript to either t or T^+ as appropriate.

To illustrate the use of this notation consider the data of Table 2.1, which gives $t_1 = 910$, $T_2^+ = 752+$, $t_3 = 1006$, and so on until $t_{12} = 641$ days. Once these survival times are ordered (ranked) in increasing magnitude, they are relabelled by $T_{(1)}^+ = 118+$, since the shortest survival time observed is censored, $t_{(2)} = 152$, $T_{(3)}^+ = 297+$ and so on until $t_{(12)} = 1006$ days. The parentheses, (.), around the subscript indicate that the data are now in rank order.

If there are tied observations then they are each given the mean rank; for example, if $t_{(4)} = t_{(5)} = t_{(6)}$, then each is relabelled $t_{(5)}$, $t_{(5)}$ and $t_{(5)}$, respectively.

2.3   SURVIVAL AT A FIXED TIME POINT

One method of describing survival data is to report the proportion of patients alive at fixed time points. Thus, for the McIllmurray and Turkie (1987) data of Figure 2.3 eight of 24 patients are known to have died by 12 months, giving a 1-year survival rate of 16/24 or 66.7%. However, this calculation presumes that the patient who is censored at 3+ months will be alive at 1 year. If, on the other hand, the patient dies before 1 year the estimate decreases to 15/24 or 62.5%.

If the same calculation were to be repeated at 2 years then seven patients with censored survival times (T^+) of less than 24 months could influence the final proportion alive at 2 years in various ways, ranging from all surviving, to all dying, at 2 years. If all survive the 2-year period then the survival rate is 12/24 (50%). In contrast, if all die the survival rate is 5/24 (21%).

Another alternative is only to use information on those patients that have reached a fixed point in the observation time. This reduced sample estimate at 1 year, for example, would exclude the patient who has a censored survival time $T^+_{(1)} = 3+$, and would give the survival rate estimate at one year as 15/23 or 65.2%. At 2 years six further patients would be removed from the denominator to give 17, of which five remain alive. The reduced sample estimate at 2 years is therefore 5/17 or 29.4%. At 3 years, five further patients are removed from the denominator to give 12, of which one remains alive. The reduced sample estimate at 3 years is therefore 1/12 or 8.3%.

In fact, dependent on the pattern of deaths and censored survival times in a data set, the reduced sample estimate of the proportion alive can *increase* with time. This is clearly an undesirable property of such an estimate since common sense tells us that the proportion alive on a particular study should not increase but will generally decrease (if only gradually) over time.

2.4   KAPLAN–MEIER OR PRODUCT-LIMIT ESTIMATE

In a clinical study a question of central interest is: what is the probability that patients will survive a certain length of time? For example, in the Stanford heart transplant data presented in Table 1.1 we may be interested in estimating the probability of a patient surviving for 1 year following heart transplant. This probability can be calculated in the following way. The probability of surviving 365 days (1 year) is the probability of surviving the 365th day having already survived the previous 364 days. Clearly one must have survived this day before one can have the possibility to survive the next day. Survival into day 365 is therefore conditional on surviving the whole of day 364. Similarly, the conditional probability of surviving for 364 days is the probability of surviving the 364th day having already survived for 363 days. This argument clearly continues for each preceding day of the one year.

In more formal terms we define

p_1 = probability of surviving for at least 1 day after transplant;
p_2 = conditional probability of surviving the second day after having survived the first day;

p_3 = conditional probability of surviving the third day after having survived the second day;

$\vdots$

p_{365} = conditional probability of surviving the 365th day after having survived day 364.

The overall probability of surviving 365 days after a heart transplant, $S(365)$, is then given by the product of these probabilities. Thus

$$S(365) = p_1 \times p_2 \times p_3 \times \ldots \times p_{364} \times p_{365}.$$

In general, the probability of survival to time t is

$$S(t) = p_1 \times p_2 \times \ldots \times p_t. \tag{2.1}$$

To calculate $S(t)$ we need to estimate each of p_1, p_2, p_3, $\ldots$, p_t. However, we can obtain an estimate of any particular one, say p_{365}, by

$$p_{365} = \frac{\text{Number of patients followed for at least 364 days and who also survive day 365}}{\text{Number of patients alive at end of day 364}}.$$

In a similar way, we can calculate for any time t

$$p_t = \frac{\text{Number of patients followed for at least } (t-1) \text{ days and who also survive day t}}{\text{Number of patients alive at end of day } (t-1)}. \tag{2.2}$$

Example

To illustrate the process we calculate p_{12} for the Dukes' C colorectal cancer data summarised in the second column of Table 2.2. It can be seen that seven patients have either died or been lost to follow-up before the 12th month; of these six have died and one is censored at 3^+ months. This leaves the number of patients at risk of death at the beginning of the 12th month as $24 - 7 = 17$. In the 12th month, however, two die but the remainder, including the censored patient with a survival of 12+ months, survive the month, leaving 15 patients alive and who will die at a later stage. Thus using equation (2.2), but now expressed in units of a month rather than days, we have

$$p_{12} = \frac{\text{Number of patients who are followed for 11 months and who survive month 12}}{\text{Number of patients alive at the end of month 11}}$$

$$= \frac{15}{17} = 0.8823.$$

Thus 88% of the patients, who survive month 11, are alive at the end month 12.

For convenience of presentation, in what follows we will assume time is measured in days but it could be seconds, minutes, hours, months or years, depending on the context.

Table 2.2 Survival data by month for the 24 patients with Dukes' C colorectal cancer randomly assigned to receive control treatment (From McIllmurray and Turkie, 1987. Reproduced by permission of *Br. Med. J.* 294: 1260 and 295: 475. (Published by BMJ Publishing Group))

Rank	Survival time t (months)	Number at risk n_t	Observed deaths d_t	$p_t = 1 - \dfrac{d_t}{n_t}$	Survival proportion $S(t)$
–	0	24	0	1.0000	1
1	3+	24	0		
2	6				
3	6	23	4	0.8261	0.8261
4	6				
5	6				
6	8	19	2	0.8947	0.7391
7	8				
8	12	17	2	0.8824	0.6522
9	12				
10	12+	15	0		
11	15+	14	0		
12	16+	13	0		
13	18+	11	0		
14	18+				
15	20	10	1	0.9000	0.5780
16	22+	9	0		
17	24	8	1	0.8750	0.5136
18	28+				
19	28+	7	0		
20	28+				
21	30	4	1	0.7500	0.3852
22	30+	3	0		
23	33+	2	0		
24	42	1	1	0.0000	0

It is convenient to think of the time, t, as denoting the start of a short time interval ending at time (t + 1). We then use n_t as the number of patients alive at the start of the interval and therefore at risk of death during that short interval. We denote the number of patients dying in the short time interval just after t as d_t. The number of patients surviving the interval is therefore $(n_t - d_t)$. This number in turn becomes the number starting interval (t + 1), which we denote by n_{t+1}. This notation enables us to write equation (2.2) as

$$p_t = \frac{(n_t - d_t)}{n_t} \qquad (2.3)$$

or,

$$p_t = 1 - \frac{d_t}{n_t}. \qquad (2.4)$$

It follows from equation (2.4) that $p_t = 1$ at times (days) when nobody dies, $d_t = 0$, since the number at risk of death at the beginning of that day is the same as the number at risk at the end of that day.

Thus the value of $S(t)$, the overall probability of survival to time t, changes only at times (days) on which at least one person dies. As a consequence, we can skip over the times (days) when there are no deaths when calculating equation (2.1).

We can rewrite equation (2.1) by using equation (2.4) as

$$S(t) = \left(1 - \frac{d_1}{n_1}\right)\left(1 - \frac{d_2}{n_2}\right)\cdots\left(1 - \frac{d_t}{n_t}\right)$$

or more briefly as

$$S(t) = \prod_t \left(1 - \frac{d_t}{n_t}\right), \tag{2.5}$$

where $\prod_t$ denotes the product of all the terms following this symbol, up to and including that of time t.

The successive overall probabilities of survival, $S(1)$, $S(2)$, ..., $S(t)$, are known as the Kaplan–Meier or product-limit estimates of survival.

It is useful to note from equation (2.1) that $S(t) = S(t-1)\, p_t$, or

$$S(t) = S(t-1)\left(1 - \frac{d_t}{n_t}\right). \tag{2.6}$$

This result enables each successive survival probability to be obtained by successive multiplication by equation (2.4). It is necessary to specify that when $t = 0$, $S(0) = 1$, i.e. all patients are assumed alive at time zero.

Example

The calculations necessary to obtain the Kaplan–Meier estimate of the survival curve using the data from the Dukes' C colorectal cancer patients of McIllmurray and Turkie (1987) are summarised in Table 2.2. We note that in this example survival time is being measured in months.

The patient survival times are first ranked, as we have indicated earlier, in terms of increasing survival. These are listed in the first column of the table. The number of patients at risk at the start, $t = 0$, is $n_0 = 24$. As time progresses, no deaths or patient losses occur until month 3, when a censored value is observed, i.e. $T_{(1)}^+ = 3^+$. As a consequence, in the next month we are not able to observe the progress of this particular patient. This leaves $n_4 = n_0 - 1 = 23$ patients potentially at risk in the following (fourth) month.

Prior to this time the number 'at risk' does not change and $n_1 = n_2 = n_3$ all equal n_0, the number of patients at risk at commencement, since the number of deaths and losses is zero. As a consequence $p_1 = p_2 = p_3 = 1$ for these months. In the months that follow $n_4 = n_5 = n_6 = 23$ remain the same, but in the sixth month the first death occurs and there are four deaths in total that month, so that $d_6 = 4$. Thus although $p_4 = p_5 = 1$, we have

$$p_6 = 1 - \frac{d_6}{n_6} = 1 - \frac{4}{23} = 0.8261.$$

By use of equation (2.5) we have therefore

$$S(6) = p_1 p_2 p_3 p_4 p_5 p_6 = 1 \times 1 \times 1 \times 1 \times 1 \times 0.8261 = 0.8261.$$

Following these deaths at 6 months, $n_7 = n_6 - d_6 = 23 - 4 = 19$ and $n_8 = 19$ also. There are then two deaths in month 8, giving $d_8 = 2$. Hence, while $p_7 = 1$, since there are no deaths in month 7, $p_8 = (1 - 2/19) = 0.8947$. From these we obtain

$$\begin{aligned}
S(8) &= p_1 p_2 p_3 p_4 p_5 p_6 p_7 p_8 \\
&= S(6)\, p_7 p_8 \\
&= 0.8261 \times 1 \times 0.8947 \\
&= 0.7391
\end{aligned}$$

In a similar way

$$\begin{aligned}
S(12) &= S(8)\, p_9 p_{10} p_{11} p_{12} \\
&= 0.7391 \times 1 \times 1 \times 1 \times 0.8824 = 0.6522
\end{aligned}$$

and so on.

The completed calculations for $S(t)$ are summarised in the last column of Table 2.2. It is worth noting that the estimate of survival beyond 42 months is zero from these data as no patient has lived (so far) beyond that time.

In contrast to the calculations in section 2.3, of survival at a fixed time point and by the reduced sample estimate, all available information, including that from those individuals with censored survival times, is included in the Kaplan–Meier estimate. For this reason the Kaplan–Meier estimate of survival is the one that should always be used.

2.5　THE SURVIVAL CURVE

The graph of $S(t)$ against the number of days, t, gives the Kaplan–Meier estimate of the survival curve and provides a useful summary of the data. $S(t)$ will start from 1 (100% of patients alive) since $S(0) = 1$, and progressively decline towards 0 (all patients have died) with time. It is plotted as a step function, since the estimated survival curve remains at a plateau between successive patient death times. It drops instantaneously at each time of death to a new level. The graph will only reach 0 if the patient with the longest observed survival time has in fact died. Were such a patient still alive then the Kaplan–Meier curve would have a plateau commencing at the time of the last death and continuing until the censored survival time of this longest surviving patient.

Example

The resulting survival curve from the calculations of Table 2.2 is shown in Figure 2.4. This curve starts at 1 and continues horizontally until the first (four) deaths at 6 months; at this time it then drops to 0.8261 and then again continues horizontally once more. Subsequently two deaths occur at month 8 and so the curve drops to 0.7391 then continues horizontally until the next death. The longest (known) survival time is for a patient who in fact died at 42 months, which is longer than any censored survival time. The Kaplan–Meier estimate is therefore zero at, and beyond, that time as previously mentioned.

We have indicated the number of patients remaining at risk as time passes under the curve at convenient (annual) time points. This information is crucial for a sensible interpretation of any survival curve. Also marked are the censored survival times, with bold vertical lines cutting the curve.

It is clear from the vertical lines that if, after a further period of observation of these patients, a death is observed amongst the (so far) censored observations, then the shape of the Kaplan–Meier curve (to the right of that point) could be substantially affected. Thus any new follow-up information on the patients with censored survival times could influence the interpretation of this study, perhaps in a substantial way.

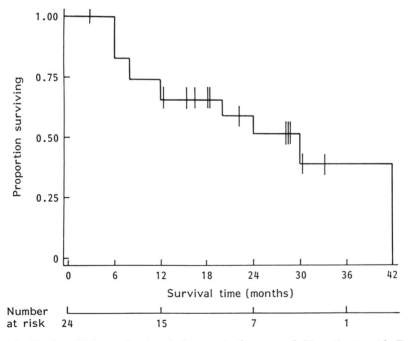

Figure 2.4 Kaplan–Meier estimate of the survival curve of 24 patients with Dukes' C colorectal cancer (From McIllmurray and Turkie, 1987. Reproduced by permission of *Br. Med. J.* 294: 1260 and 295: 475. (Published by BMJ Publishing Group))

Example from the literature

Samanta *et al.* (1991) reported on the duration of intramuscular gold therapy in 78 patients with rheumatoid arthritis. They calculated the Kaplan–Meier 'survival' curve which is shown in Figure 2.5.

For these patients the first critical event is the start of gold therapy for their rheumatoid arthritis and the second critical event (endpoint) is cessation of this therapy for whatever reason. From the survival curve they estimate that the proportion continuing with gold therapy at 10 years (120 months) is approximately 50%. This can be verified by moving vertically from 120 months on the time scale until the Kaplan–Meier curve is cut and then moving horizontally to cut the S(t) axis. This cut occurs at 0.5 and so we can write S(120) = 0.5. The authors give no indication in their text figure of the numbers at risk (here patients continuing on treatment) with time and do not indicate the censored gold therapy duration times. We note that in this context the censored values indicate patients who are still continuing on gold therapy.

In certain circumstances for presentation purposes a graph of [1 − S(t)], rather than S(t), is plotted against t to give the cumulative death curve. Such a plot can be observed from the S(t) plot by first turning the page over and holding the upside-down page to the light. This method of plotting is sometimes chosen if the outcome event is relatively rare or is of benefit to the patient. Thus the healing of an ulcer, achieving a pregnancy if you are being treated for infertility, and discharge (fit) from hospital are all examples of successful outcomes.

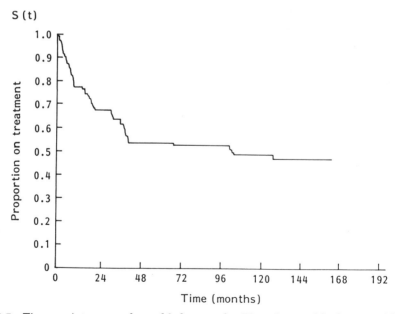

Figure 2.5 Time on intramuscular gold therapy for 78 patients with rheumatoid arthritis (From Samanta *et al.*, 1991. Gold therapy in rheumatoid arthritis, *Lancet*, 338, 642, © by The Lancet Ltd)

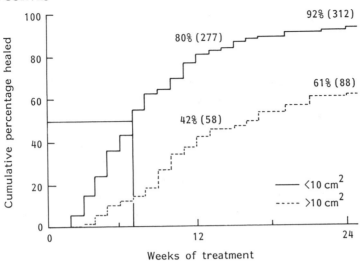

Figure 2.6 Cumulative rate of healing of limbs with venous ulceration of area less than or greater than 10 cm² (after Moffatt *et al.*, 1992)

Example from the literature

Moffatt *et al.* (1992) calculated the Kaplan–Meier cumulative rates, $1 - S(t)$, of healing of limbs with venous ulceration for different groups of patients. The cumulative healing rate for those 349 patients whose ulcers have areas of less than 10 cm² at presentation is shown by the solid line in Figure 2.6. Approximately 50% of these ulcers have healed by 7 weeks. The authors quote the numbers of patients observed up to and including 12 and 24 weeks, and so the remaining numbers at risk of 72 and 37 can be calculated. We note that censored observations are not indicated, although presenting these is not always easy to do in an uncluttered way when there are many censored observations. Those patients with large ulcers (>10 cm²), denoted by the hatched line in Figure 2.6, appear to heal more slowly, as one might expect.

2.6   MEDIAN SURVIVAL TIME

If there are no censored observations, for example all the patients have died on a clinical trial, then the median survival time, M, is estimated by the middle observation of the ranked survival times, $t_{(1)}, t_{(2)}, \ldots, t_{(n)}$ if the number of observations, n, is odd, and by the average of $t_{(n/2)}$ and $t_{(n/2+1)}$ if n is even, i.e.

$$M = t_{([n+1]/2)} \text{ if n is odd}$$
$$= \frac{1}{2}\left[t_{(n/2)} + t_{(n/2+1)}\right] \text{ if n is even.} \qquad (2.7)$$

In the presence of censored survival times the median survival is estimated by first calculating the Kaplan–Meier survival curve, then finding the value of M that satisfies the equation

$$S(M) = 0.5. \tag{2.8}$$

This can be done by extending a horizontal line from $S(t) = 0.5$ (or 50%) on the vertical axis of the Kaplan–Meier survival curve, until the actual curve is met, then moving vertically down from that point to cut the horizontal time axis at M, the median survival time.

A parallel calculation, to estimate the proportion continuing on gold therapy at 120 months or 10 years in the study by Samanta *et al.* (1991), was described earlier.

It should be emphasised that the estimate of the median does not use the individual values of the data items, except those immediately surrounding M, but only their ranks. One consequence of this is that the associated standard error of the median, SE(M), is large and therefore statistical tests based on the median are insensitive.

Example from the literature

The median time from the first CD4 cell count below 200/μl to the development of AIDS in HIV-infected men is given as 651 days by van Griensven *et al.* (1991). For these men the first event is a CD4 cell count below 200/μl and the subsequent (end-point) event is the development of AIDS some time later. The corresponding Kaplan–Meier survival curve is shown in Figure 2.7 and the hatched lines indicate how the median is obtained.

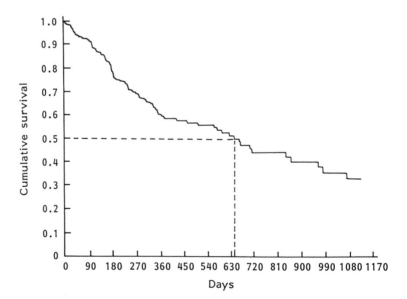

Figure 2.7 Probability of freedom from AIDS (expressed as survival) among 161 homosexual men with CD4 count below 200/μl (From van Griensven *et al.*, 1991. Expansion of AIDS case definition. *Lancet*, 338, 1012–1013, © by The Lancet Ltd)

Example from the literature

Khawaja *et al.* (1988) estimate the median infusion survival time as 127 hours in 170 patients from a general surgical unit randomised to receive transdermal glyceryl trinitrate. The object of the therapy was to increase the length of time of the infusion. In contrast, the median infusion survival time in the 170 patients randomised to a placebo infusion was only 74 hours.

In a similar way the median survival time of the patients with Dukes' C colorectal cancer is estimated from Figure 2.4 as 30 months. The 7-week median healing time of the limb ulcers, reported by Moffatt *et al.* (1992), of less than 10 cm^2 at presentation was indicated earlier. This latter example uses the cumulative estimate of the death curve, $1 - S(t)$, but the median is unchanged, since $[1 - S(t)] = 0.5$ at the same time point as $S(t) = 0.5$. The median healing of those ulcers >10 cm^2 is approximately 20 weeks.

2.7 INTERPRETATION OF THE SURVIVAL CURVE

The Kaplan–Meier estimate of the survival curve is the best description of times to death of a group of patients using all the data currently available. If all the patients have died before the data are analysed the estimate is exactly the same as the proportion of survivors plotted against time. In this case the proportions are plotted at each death time and the size of the downward part of the step will be $1/n_0$ at every death time, where n_0 is the initial number of patients under observation, unless there are tied observations when two or more patients die with the same survival time. In this circumstance the step down will be that multiple of $1/n_0$. Each step starts at each successive death time and the process continues until the final death, which will have the longest survival time.

The overall survival curve is much more reliable than the individually observed conditional survival probabilities, p_t, of which it is composed. Nevertheless spurious (large) jumps or (long) flat sections may sometimes appear. These are most likely to occur if the proportion of censored observations is large and in areas in the extreme right of the curve when the number of patients still alive and being followed up may be relatively small.

Example

In the data of van Griensven *et al.* (1991), describing the probability of remaining free of AIDS after the first CD4 count below 200/μl, there is a section beyond 720 days in Figure 2.7 when the steps are deeper than in other sections of the curve. There is also a suggestion of some levelling off (plateauing) beyond this time, with relatively long gaps between successive events.

Both of these features may be spurious. The suggestion of a plateau may be explained by the relatively few subjects still on follow-up and so far without AIDS at and beyond 2 years. Thus there is very little information in this part of the curve. The rather larger steps here may result from a single patient developing AIDS at this stage, amongst the few that have been followed to that date.

Other spurious features can also occur, thus the apparent rapid drop close to 180 days (6 months) may not be that the rate of development of AIDS is faster around this period of time but is more likely to be a feature of prearranged clinic visits. Thus if individuals are being tested for AIDS at a prearranged 6-month visit, and are then found to have AIDS on examination, it is the clinic visit date that is recorded as the date of (proven) onset of AIDS. However, the true onset of the, as yet, undetected AIDS is likely to have occurred at an earlier date.

As indicated earlier, a guide to the reliability of different portions of the survival curve can be obtained by recording the number of patients at risk at various stages beneath the time axis of the survival curve, as we illustrated in Figure 2.4. The 'number at risk' is defined as the number of patients who are known to be alive at that timepoint and therefore have not yet died nor have been censored before the timepoint. At time zero, which is the time of entry of patients into the study, all patients are at risk and hence the number 'at risk' recorded beneath $t = 0$ is n_0, the number of patients entered into the study. The patient numbers obviously diminish as time elapses, both because of deaths and censoring, and thereby their number also indicates the diminishing reliability of the Kaplan–Meier estimate of $S(t)$ with increasing t.

It is difficult to judge precisely when the right-hand tail of the survival curve becomes unreliable. However, as a rule of thumb, the curve can be particularly unreliable when the number of patients remaining at risk is less than 15. The width of the confidence intervals (see section 2.8), calculated at these and other timepoints, will help to decide this in a particular circumstance. Nevertheless, it is not uncommon to see the value of $S(t)$, corresponding to the final plateau, being quoted for example for patients with cancer as the 'cure' rate—especially if the plateau is long. This can be seriously misleading as the rate will almost certainly be reduced with further patient follow-up. Clearly, if there are no censored observations preceding the end of a plateau, then the plateau will not disappear with more patient follow-up. Even in such cases the plateau should be interpreted with considerable caution.

2.8   CONFIDENCE INTERVALS FOR S(t)

We have indicated earlier that confidence intervals (CI) calculated at key points along the Kaplan–Meier survival curve will give an indication of the reliability of the estimates at those points. These can be calculated for the timepoint of interest using the usual format for CIs of equation (1.4) by assuming a Normal distribution for the Kaplan–Meier estimates, $S(t)$. Thus, the 95% CI at time t is

$$S(t) - 1.96 \, SE[S(t)] \quad \text{to} \quad S(t) + 1.96 SE[S(t)]. \qquad (2.9)$$

There are several ways in which an estimate of $SE[S(t)]$ can be obtained. We first review three widely used methods and then present the transformation method, which is our recommended approach.

GREENWOOD'S METHOD

One estimate for SE[S(t)] is that given by Greenwood (1926), which is

$$SE_{Gr}[S(t)] = S(t)\left(\sum_{j=0}^{t-1} \frac{d_j}{n_j(n_j - d_j)}\right)^{1/2}. \tag{2.10}$$

Here d_j is the number of deaths on day j and n_j is the number of patients alive and on follow-up at the beginning of day j. Just as we noted, prior to equation (2.5) when describing the Kaplan–Meier calculations, equation (2.10) too is only affected on days that at least one death occurs.

Example

To illustrate the calculation of $SE_{Gr}[S(t)]$ and the corresponding 95% CI we use the data from the patients with Dukes' C colorectal cancer summarised in Table 2.2. For example, at $t = 12$ months the Kaplan–Meier estimate of the proportion alive is $S(12) = 0.6522$ or 65%, and since there are four deaths at 6 months and two deaths at 8 months prior to this time, we have from equation (2.10) that

$$SE_{Gr}[S(12)] = 0.6522\left[\frac{4}{23(23 - 4)} + \frac{2}{19(19 - 2)}\right]^{1/2}$$

$$= 0.6522\ (0.009153 + 0.006192)^{1/2}$$

$$= 0.6522 \times 0.12387$$

$$= 0.0808$$

We note here that, although $n_0 = 24$ patients were recruited to this study, one of these is censored at $T^+ = 3^+$ months before any death occurs. Consequently the number at risk before any death is reduced to $n_0 - 1 = 23$, which is the figure used in the above calculation.

The 95% CI for S(12), using the SE estimated by $SE_{Gr}[S(12)]$, is therefore from $0.6522 - 1.96 \times 0.0808 = 0.4938$ to $0.6522 + 1.96 \times 0.0808 = 0.8106$. The wide CI, of 49% to 81% survival, gives some indication of how little information is available on the survival rate of these patients at this time. CIs at 2 and 3 years (say) will be correspondingly wider than these as the SE increases with time.

Example from the literature

Hankey *et al.* (1991) calculate the Kaplan–Meier survival curve of 99 patients following retinal infarction without prior stroke. Their survival curve is shown in Figure 2.8 and illustrates the 95% CI calculated at each year. The width of these intervals widens with successive years, reflecting the reduced number of patients at risk as time passes.

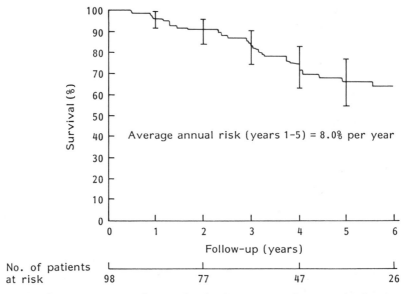

Figure 2.8 Kaplan–Meier survival curve for the first 6 years after retinal infarction. Bars at each year are 95% confidence intervals (From Hankey *et al.*, 1991. Reproduced by permission of *Br. Med. J.* 302: 499–504.)

PETO'S METHOD

Greenwood's formula is only accurate for large numbers of subjects alive at the time point under consideration and so strictly was not very appropriate in our example. In particular, the Greenwood method tends to underestimate the SE, especially in the tail of the survival curve, so that its use only provides a guide to the minimum width of the corresponding CI. A more reliable estimate of the SE and one which is easier to calculate is given by Peto (1984). This is given by

$$SE_P[S(t)] = \left\{ \frac{S(t)[1 - S(t)]}{R_t} \right\}^{1/2} \tag{2.11}$$

where R_t is the number of patients recruited to the trial minus the number censored by the time under consideration. Thus $R_t = n_0 - c_t$, where c_t is the number of patients censored before time t. R_t is sometimes termed the 'effective' sample size.

If there are no censored observations before this timepoint then this SE is the same as that for the SE given in Table 1.2. In our context we replace p by S(t), thus

$$SE = \sqrt{\{S(t)[1 - S(t)]/n_0\}} \tag{2.12}$$

If we use equation (2.11) in place of equation (2.10) with the data from the colorectal cancer patients we have $R_{12} = 24 - 1 = 23$ and therefore $SE_p[S(12)] = [0.6522 \times (1 - 0.6522)/23]^{1/2} = 0.0993$. Thus, in this example, SE_p is a little larger than that given by the Greenwood (SE_{Gr}). The corresponding 95% CI for S(12) of 0.4575 to 0.8468 or 46% to 85% is therefore a little wider than that of the previous calculation.

It should be emphasised that the CIs just calculated are approximate and have equal width above and below the estimate S(t). The technically 'correct' CIs should only be symmetric about S(t) when S(t) is close to 0.5. However, these approximations will usually be satisfactory provided S(t) is neither close to 1 or close to 0, i.e. near the beginning or end of the Kaplan–Meier curve. In such situations the CI is restricted by, for example, the horizontal time axis as negative values of the lower confidence limit are not possible. Similarly, values within the CI beyond unity (100% survival) are not possible.

ROTHMAN'S METHOD

A method of calculating CIs taking into account the constraints of 0 and 1 on the values of S(t) has been suggested by Rothman (1978). In essence this method is similar to the 'effective sample size' introduced when describing the Peto method.

Once S(t) and R_t are determined then these are used in tables of the so-called exact CIs for a proportion in the following way. To use these tables you need to specify n, the number of subjects and r, the number of responses amongst these subjects, which together provide the estimate of the proportion of responders $p = r/n$. In our context $p = S(t)$, $n = R_t$ and $r = R_tS(t)$. The value of r calculated in this way will not usually be an integer and therefore in practice is rounded to the nearest whole number. The values of r and n calculated are then referred to the tables of the exact CIs given by, for example, Lentner (1991, pp. 89–102). These CIs will not be symmetric about S(t) unless $S(t) = 0.5$ exactly.

Example

For the patients with Dukes' C colorectal cancer we estimate that $S(12) = 0.6522$ and $n = R_{12} = 23$. These give $r = R_{12}S(12) = 23 \times 0.6522 = 15.00$. In this example, r is an exact integer but this is because there are no censored observations between the times of 6 and 12 months. Reference to the tables cited above with $n = 23$ and $r = 15$ gives a 95% CI as 0.43 to 0.84 or 43% to 84%.

TRANSFORMATION METHOD

Another alternative method of calculating a CI, and as we mentioned earlier the method we recommend, is to transform S(t) onto a scale which more closely follows a Normal distribution. Thus it can be shown that $\log\{-\log[S(t)]\}$ has an approximately Normal distribution, with SE given by

$$SE_{Tr}[S(t)] = \frac{\left[\sum_{j=0}^{t-1} \frac{d_j}{n_j(n_j - d_j)}\right]^{1/2}}{\left[-\sum_{j=0}^{t-1} \log\left(\frac{n_j - d_j}{n_j}\right)\right]}. \tag{2.13}$$

Use of equation (2.9) then gives, on this transformed scale, a 95% CI of

$$\log\{-\log[S(t)]\} - 1.96SE_{Tr} \quad \text{to} \quad \log\{-\log[S(t)]\} + 1.96SE_{Tr}. \quad (2.14)$$

To return to the untransformed scale we have to antilog the lower and upper values of this CI given by equation (2.14), take the negative of these and then antilog again. The result of this quite involved process is summarised by

$$S(t)^{\exp(+1.96SE_{Tr})} \quad \text{to} \quad S(t)^{\exp(-1.96SE_{Tr})}. \quad (2.15)$$

Note the signs attached to 1.96 in equation (2.15) are correct.

Example

Repeating the earlier example for $S(12) = 0.6522$, we have from equation (2.13), that

$$SE = \sqrt{\left[\frac{4}{23(23-4)} + \frac{2}{19(19-2)}\right] \bigg/ \left[-\log\left(\frac{23-4}{23}\right) - \log\left(\frac{19-2}{19}\right)\right]}$$

$$= \sqrt{(0.014345)/(+0.191055 + 0.111226)}$$

$$= 0.4098.$$

From this $\exp(+1.96SE_{Tr}) = 2.2327$, $\exp(-1.96SE_{Tr}) = 0.4479$ and finally the 95% CI is $S(t)^{2.2327} = 0.3851$ to $S(t)^{0.4479} = 0.8258$, or 39% to 83%.

This CI is not symmetric around $S(12) = 0.6522$ (65%) and is wider than that for all the methods presented earlier.

2.9   CONFIDENCE INTERVAL FOR THE WHOLE CURVE

It is possible to calculate a CI about the whole Kaplan–Meier survival curve rather than just at fixed and perhaps rather arbitrary points along it. Although we do not describe the method here, as it is not used very often, it is described in some detail by Harris and Albert (1991, Ch. 2) in their text, which also includes a rather necessary computer program on diskette for the calculation of such confidence curves.

Example from the literature

Harris and Albert (1991) calculate the 95% CI curves around the Kaplan–Meier survival curve for patients diagnosed with rectal cancer. These are shown in Figure 2.9 and indicate how much uncertainty there is with respect to the true path of the survival curve of patients within that study.

2.10   CONFIDENCE INTERVAL FOR A MEDIAN

Example from the literature

As indicated in Figure 2.7 the median time in the development of AIDS given by van Griensven *et al.* (1991) in their study was 651 days (21 months) with a 95% CI

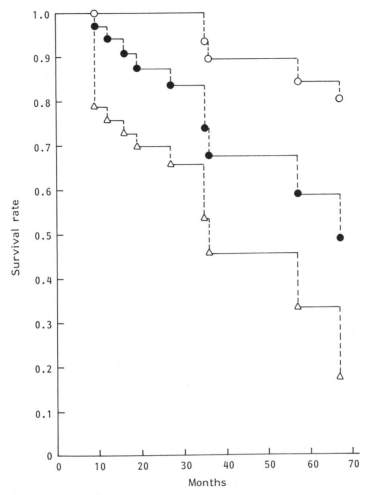

Figure 2.9 The 95% confidence intervals around the whole Kaplan–Meier estimate of the survival curve for patients with rectal cancer (From Harris and Albert, 1991. Reproduced by permission of *Survivorship Analysis for Clinical Studies*, Marcel Dekker, New York, p. 46)

of 429 to 865 days or 14 to 32 months. This leaves considerable uncertainty with respect to the median's true value.

The calculations required for the CI of a median are quite complicated and an explanation of how these are derived is complex. A clear description of the technical aspects is given by Collett (1994). He gives an expression for the SE of the median as:

$$SE_{Median} = SE_{Gr}[S(M)]\{(t_{Small} - t_{Large})/[S(t_{Large}) - S(t_{Small})]\} \qquad (2.16)$$

where t_{Small} is the smallest observed survival time from the Kaplan–Meier curve for which $S(t)$ is less than or equal to 0.45, while t_{Large} is the largest survival observed survival time from the Kaplan–Meier curve for which $S(t)$ is greater than 0.55.

Example

If we use the Kaplan–Meier estimate of the survival time of patients with Dukes' C colorectal cancer then from Figure 2.4 the median $M = 30$ months approximately. Reading from Table 2.2 at $S(t)$ less than 0.45 gives $t_{Small} = 30$ months also and for $S(t)$ greater than 0.55 we have $t_{Large} = 20$ months.

We then need an estimate of the SE of $S(t)$ which is

$$SE_{Gr}[S(30)] = 0.5 \left[\frac{4}{23(23-4)} + \frac{2}{19(19-2)} + \frac{2}{17(17-2)} + \frac{1}{10(10-1)} + \frac{1}{8(8-1)} \right]^{1/2}$$

$$= 0.5 (0.009153 + 0.006192 + 0.007843 + 0.011111 + 0.017857)^{1/2}$$

$$= 0.5 \times 0.228377 = 0.114188.$$

Therefore

$$SE_{Median} = 0.114188 \times [(30 - 20)/(0.5780 - 0.3852)]$$
$$= 0.114188 \times 51.8672 = 5.92.$$

The 95% CI is

$$M - 1.96 SE_{Gr}[SE_{Median}] \qquad \text{to} \qquad M + 1.96 SE_{Gr}[SE_{Median}] \qquad (2.17)$$

Thus, for our example, this is $30 - 11.60 = 18.40$ to $30 + 11.60 = 41.60$ months or approximately 18 to 42 months.

However, we must caution against the uncritical use of this method for such small data sets, since as we have indicated before the value of SE_{Gr} is unreliable in such circumstances, and also the values of t_{Small} and t_{Large} will be poorly determined.

2.11   THE HAZARD RATE

In many situations it is important to know how the risk of a particular outcome changes with time. For example, it is well known that infant mortality is highest in the few days following birth and thereafter declines very rapidly. Similarly, there is usually additional (short-term) risk following some medical procedures.

Example from the literature

Farley *et al.* (1992) show how the risk of pelvic inflammatory disease (PID) associated with the use of an intrauterine device (IUD) for contraceptive purposes is at its greatest in the immediate post-insertion period. This risk reduced from 9.4 to 1.4 per 1000 woman years after the first 20 days and remained at 1.4 per 1000 for up to 8 years. Their PID incidence rates are shown in Figure 2.10.

The risk or hazard rate can be estimated, within specific time intervals, by dividing the total period of survival into time segments, counting the number of events arising in the segment and dividing by the number of patients at risk during that segment. When the unit of time is a day, it is the probability of the event occurring within the (next) day, given that you have survived to that day. In a

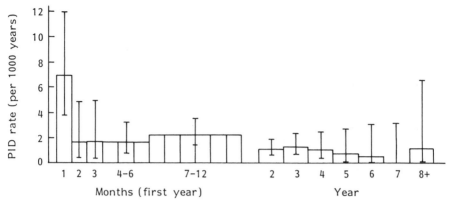

Figure 2.10 PID incidence and 95% confidence intervals by time since insertion of an IUD (From Farley *et al.*, 1992, Intrauterine devices and pelvic inflammatory disease: an international perspective. *Lancet*, 339, 785–788. © by The Lancet Ltd)

survival time context the hazard rate can be interpreted as the risk of dying on that particular day. In this framework if the time segment is short it is sometimes referred to as the instantaneous death rate.

Example

We illustrate the idea of the hazard rate by calculating the annual (i.e. yearly) hazard rate (h), for the data of Table 2.2. We first calculate the total months of exposure for all patients during the first year. Six patients (d_1) died during the first year: four at 6 months and two at 8 months. We define their total exposure during the first year as f_1, where

$$f_1 = (4 \text{ patients} \times 6 \text{ months}) + (2 \text{ patients} \times 8 \text{ months})$$
$$= 40 \text{ months of exposure.}$$

Of the patients alive, one was censored at 3 months while 17 survive the 12 months. The exposure time contributed by these 18 patients is F_1, where

$$F_1 = (1 \times 3) + (17 \times 12)$$
$$= 207 \text{ months of exposure.}$$

The total exposure during the first year for the 24 patients is therefore $f_1 + F_1 = 40 + 207$ months = 247 months. The hazard rate for the first year is $h_1 = d_1/(f_1 + F_1) = 6/247 = 0.02429$ per month. On an annual basis this is $0.02429 \times 12 = 0.29$ or 29 per 100 person years of exposure for the first year.

For the second year, there are two deaths at 12 months (we are assuming here that these patients just survived the first year but died immediately after) and a death at 20 months, hence $d_2 = 3$ deaths in the second interval. These three deaths therefore contribute $f_2 = (2 \times 0) + (1 \times 8) = 8$ months of exposure within this second interval. Censored values occur at 12+, 15+, 16+, 18+, 18+ and 22+ months. These six patients therefore contribute 0, 3, 4, 6, 6 and 10 months or a total of 29 months to the second interval. There are also eight patients who survive beyond the second interval and who together contribute $8 \times 12 = 96$ months to the exposure. Collectively these 14 patients contribute $F_2 = 29 + 96 = 125$ months of exposure within the second interval. The total exposure is therefore, $f_2 + F_2 = 8 + 145 = 153$ months, and the hazard is $h_2 = d_2/(f_2 + F_2) = 3/153 = 0.019608$ per month. On an annual basis this is 0.24 or 24 per 100 person years for the second year. Similar calculations give $h_3 = 2/33 = 0.06061$ and $h_4 = 1/6 = 0.16667$ per month or 73 and 200 per 100 person years, for the third and fourth years, respectively.

In this example, the values we obtain for h_1 and h_2 depend rather critically on how we deal with the deaths at the boundaries of the intervals. Such problems only arise if there are several tied events at the boundaries. In the above example, two deaths at 12 months occur at the break of the interval. If we ascribe these deaths to the first interval then $h_1 = d_1/(f_1 + F_1) = 8/247 = 0.03239$ per month. On an annual basis this is 0.39 or 39 per 100 person years for the first year. These two deaths will not of course now occur in the second interval but the death at 24 months is now counted in the interval. Consequently, $d_2 = 2$ and $h_2 = d_2/(f_2 + F_2) = 2/153 = 0.01307$ per month. On an annual basis this is 0.16 or 16 per 100 person years.

The above hazards of 29, 24, 73 and 200 per 100 person years are sometimes expressed as 29%, 24%, 73% and 200% respectively, although they are strictly not percentages.

With such a small data set we should not be too surprised at the above changes. They do emphasise, however, that survival time is best recorded in small time units so that tied observations can be avoided if possible and events assigned to the appropriate interval without ambiguity.

In chapter 3, equation (3.4), we discuss the situation when we can assume that the hazard is constant, i.e. the rate of death in successive intervals remains the same.

Example from the literature

Stephens *et al.* (1994) calculated the daily hazard obtained from data on more than 2000 patients with small cell lung cancer. These data are shown in Figure 2.11 and show that except for a period between 8 and 14 days from start of treatment the daily hazard appears to be approximately constant. Outside of this time period there appear to be random fluctuations, which are to be expected because the 1-day unit of time is small. The authors suggest that the increased hazard rates during the 8 to 14 day period may be due to a treatment-induced mortality.

Example from the literature

Fisher *et al.* (1991) calculated the hazard for each year following treatment for breast cancer. They reported the average hazard for ipsilateral tumour recurrence— reappearance of a tumour in the same breast—for the women having lumpectomy as 6.6% while for those who received radiotherapy in addition to lumpectomy the hazard was 1.4%. The annual hazards for 10 successive years for the two patient groups are shown in Figure 2.12.

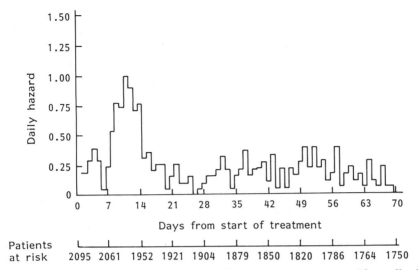

Figure 2.11 Estimated daily hazard from start of treatment in patients with small cell lung cancer (after Stephens *et al.*, 1994)

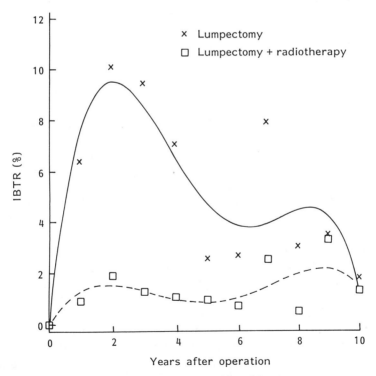

Figure 2.12 Smoothed yearly hazard plots for ipsilateral breast tumour recurrence (IBTR) (From Fisher *et al.*, 1991. Significance of ipsilateral breast tumour recurrence after lumpectomy. *Lancet*, 338, 327–331. © by The Lancet Ltd)

This graph illustrates an approximately constant hazard in the 10 postoperative years for those women who received lumpectomy plus radiotherapy (XRT). In contrast, the hazard for those who had lumpectomy without XRT appears to be much higher initially, but then declines to levels similar to those who received XRT, during and after the fifth postoperative year. The authors do not explain the method of smoothing the hazards shown in the figure.

The hazard rate is also discussed in relation to the exponential distribution in section 3.2 and the Pearl rate in section 11.1.

2.12   FOLLOW-UP MATURITY

As discussed earlier and in chapter 1, in any study with a survival-type endpoint there will usually be a mixture of subjects in which the critical event has been observed and those in which it has not. As a consequence it is often useful to have a measure which will help to give a brief summary of the maturity of the data being analysed. Mature data are those in which most of the events that can be anticipated have been observed. Although the numbers at risk at various stages along the Kaplan–Meier survival curve and the indication of the censored data on these curves together with SEs at specific time points (see for example Figure 2.4), do fulfil this purpose to some extent, they do not give a concise means of assessing follow-up maturity. Simple summaries which have been suggested for this purpose include the median follow-up time of those individuals still alive, together with the minimum and maximum follow-up times of these individuals.

Example

In Table 2.2 there are 12 surviving from the 24 patients with Dukes' C colorectal cancer of McIllmurray and Turkie (1987), with corresponding ordered censored survival times of 3+, 12+, 15+, 16+, 18+, 18+, 22+, 28+, 28+, 28+, 30+ and 33+ months. Thus 50% of the potential events have not yet been observed, which may suggest the data are not very mature. The minimum follow-up of those still alive is 3 months, the median follow-up is $(18 + 22)/2 = 20$ months and the maximum follow-up is 33 months. The median rather than mean follow-up time is chosen since, as already indicated, the distributions of survival time data are usually skewed.

A more complete graphical method has been suggested in which follow-up information on all patients, both dead and alive, is used. The first step is to construct a Kaplan–Meier 'follow-up' curve. To do this, we label those patients who have 'died' as actually being 'censored' on their date of death, and those patients who are still alive as having an 'event' on the date they were censored. That is, we reverse the censoring. The reason for this is that since our principal attention is now on a different 'endpoint', that of follow-up, those patients who have died could theoretically have provided more follow-up, while those who have actually been censored have reached the end of their follow-up (as far as the current data set is concerned). The estimated median follow-up can be read off the curves in the same way as median survival.

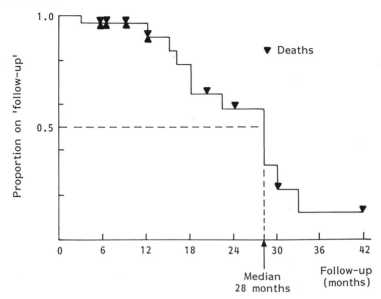

Figure 2.13 The Kaplan–Meier 'follow-up curve' for patients with Dukes' C colorectal cancer

Example

The Kaplan–Meier follow-up curve for the 24 patients with colorectal cancer is shown in Figure 2.13. From this we obtain the median follow-up as 28 months, which contrasts with the 20 months given earlier using the alive patients only.

We should point out, however, that such an approach, and indeed the whole concept of measuring median follow-up by whatever method, has been criticised by Shuster (1991), who states: 'median follow-up is not a valid or useful scientific term'. He gives examples of how it can be misleading, particularly since it can be low with excellent follow-up or high with poor follow-up.

Nevertheless, although it may have its drawbacks when describing only one group, the graphical method just described may have greater use when comparing two or more groups, as we discuss in chapter 4.

2.13 ACTUARIAL METHOD

In some situations the survival time may not be recorded as precisely as may be possible and the corresponding critical event is merely noted to have occurred in a particular time interval. Thus McIllmurray and Turkie (1987) report their data to the nearest month. For illustrative purposes we will suppose that they had recorded deaths in 6-month intervals, in which case their data would take the form of Table 2.3. In this situation we would have to take 6 months as our 'unit' of time, and the survival curve and table calculated are called the life-table or actuarial estimates.

Table 2.3 Actuarial estimate of the survival for the data from McIllmurray and Turkie (1987). Reproduced by permission of Br. Med. J. 294: 1260 and 295: 475. But grouped in 6-month intervals (we assume that those who were recorded as died at 6 months died within the first 6 months)

Interval	Time period	d_j	c_j	n_j	n_j'	$(n_j' - d_j)/n_j'$	$S_{Actuarial}(t)$
1	0–	4	1	24	23.5	0.8298	0.8298
2	6–	4	0	19	19.0	0.7895	0.6551
3	12–	0	3	15	13.5	1.0000	0.6551
4	18–	2	3	12	10.5	0.5303	0.3474
5	24–	1	3	7	5.5	0.8182	0.2843
6	30–	0	2	3	2.0	1.0000	0.2843
7	36–	1	0	1	1.0	0.0000	0.0000

The actuarial estimate of the survival table is obtained by first dividing the period of observation into a series of time intervals. These intervals need not necessarily be of equal length, although they usually are. Suppose that the jth of the m such intervals, $j = 1, 2, \ldots, m$, extends from time t_j' to t_{j+1}', and let d_j and c_j denote the number of deaths and the number of censored survival times, respectively, in this time interval.

Also let n_j be the number of individuals who are alive, and therefore at risk of death, at the start of the jth interval. We now make the assumption that the censoring process is such that the censored survival times occur uniformly throughout the interval j, so that the average number of individuals who are at risk during this interval is

$$n_j' = n_j - c_j/2. \qquad (2.18)$$

This assumption is sometimes known as the actuarial assumption. In the jth interval, the probability of death can be estimated by d_j/n_j'. Now consider the probability that an individual survives beyond time t_k', $k = 1, 2, \ldots, m$, i.e. until some time after the start of the kth interval and through each of the $k - 1$ preceding intervals, and so the actuarial estimate of the survival is given by

$$S_{Actuarial}(t) = \prod_{j=1}^{k} \left(\frac{n_j' - d_j}{n_j'} \right) \qquad (2.19)$$

for $t_k' < t < t_{k+1}'$, $k = 1, 2, \ldots, m$. This is exactly the same form as equation (2.5). The estimated probability of surviving until the start of the first interval, t_1', is of course unity, while the estimated probability of surviving beyond the end of the last interval, t_{m+1}', is zero. A graphical estimate of the survival curve will then be a step-function with constant values of the curve within each time interval.

Example

To illustrate the computation of the actuarial estimate, consider the data of Table 2.3 on the survival times of patients with Dukes' C colorectal cancer. The survival

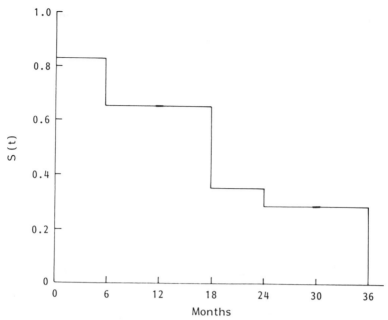

Figure 2.14   Actuarial estimate of the survival curve for the data of Table 2.3

times are first grouped to give the number of patients who die, d_j, and the number who are censored, c_j, in each of the 6-month periods of the study.

The number at risk of death at the start of each of these intervals, n_j, is then computed, together with the adjusted number at risk, n_j'. Finally, the probability of survival through each interval is estimated, from which the estimated survival curve is obtained using equation (2.19). The calculations are shown in Table 2.3, in which the time period is given in months, and a graph of the life table estimate of the survival curve is shown in Figure 2.14. The form of the estimated survival function obtained using this method is sensitive to the choice of the intervals used in its construction.

2.14   OTHER FORMS OF CENSORING

The censoring that we deal with in this book is the most common in human studies and has been called type III censoring (Lee, 1992). Lee describes two other types of censoring that may occur. In type I censoring, which is common in animal studies, all animals are recruited to the study on the same day (since they do not volunteer or need to give consent). On that day they may all receive some intervention (the first event) and then they are all followed for a fixed period of time in order to observe the critical (endpoint) events if and when they occur. Those animals who do not experience this event within the fixed time period all have the same censored time, which is the duration of the experiment.

In contrast, for type II censoring one waits until a predetermined proportion of the animals have experienced the critical event. At that time, all other animals will have censored survival times which again will usually all be equal.

Both these types of censoring mechanisms change into type III censoring if an animal is lost to follow-up for reasons beyond the experimenter's control before the 'end' of the experiment. For example, in experiments with mice it is not unknown for them to escape or (perhaps) be eaten by a colleague!

2.15 TECHNICAL DETAILS

It is convenient to think of the survival times in a particular context of having a distribution. In Figure 2.15 we sketch the form that this might take. We can then interpret S(t), for any given time t, as the proportion of the total area under the curve, to the left of t. The total area under the curve is unity. If we denote the height of the distribution at the particular time by $\phi(t)$, then $\phi(t)$ is known as the probability density function. We introduced earlier (section 2.11) the hazard rate which may vary with time and which we denote by h(t). There are mathematical relationships between S(t), $\phi(t)$ and h(t) which we now describe.

The distributional form of survival times may be presented by either the survivor function (previously called the survival curve) S(t), the hazard function h(t), or the probability density function $\phi(t)$.

The probability density function is the probability of a death occurring at time t which is contained in a very small time interval between τ and $\tau + \Delta\tau$. That is

$$\phi(t) = \lim_{\Delta\tau \to 0} \left\{ \frac{\text{Prob[death in interval}(\tau, \tau + \Delta\tau)]}{\Delta\tau} \right\}. \qquad (2.20)$$

The survival function, S(t) = Prob (individual survives longer than time t). This is the probability of surviving at least as long as t, which is 1 minus the integral of $\phi(t)$ up to time t, i.e.

$$S(t) = 1 - \int_0^t \phi(u) \, du. \qquad (2.21)$$

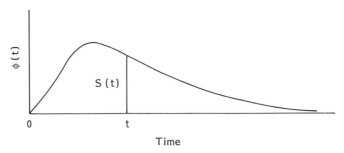

Figure 2.15   Distribution of survival times

Finally, the hazard function is the instantaneous failure rate at t, which is the probability of dying in the next small interval, having already survived to the beginning of the interval. This is defined as

$$h(t) = \underset{\Delta \tau \to 0}{\text{limit}} \left[\frac{\text{Prob}(\tau < t < \tau + \Delta \tau \mid \tau \leqslant t)}{\Delta \tau} \right]. \qquad (2.22)$$

The hazard and survival functions can be expressed in terms of each other, since

$$\phi(t) = \frac{d}{dt} [1 - S(t)]$$

and

$$h(t) = \frac{\phi(t)}{S(t)} = -\frac{d}{dt} [\log S(t)]. \qquad (2.23)$$

The hazard, survival and probability density functions are therefore alternative forms of describing the distribution of survival times. The survival function is most useful for comparing the survival progress of two or more patient groups. The hazard function, since it is an instantaneous measure, gives a more useful graphical description of the risk of failure at any time point t. It is not necessarily always increasing or decreasing.

3 The Exponential and Weibull Distributions

Summary

This chapter describes two parametric models which are often useful with survival data. We first introduce the exponential distribution, which can be used if we can assume that the hazard rate is constant within a particular group of individuals. Graphical techniques to help assess the validity of the assumption of a constant hazard rate are presented. In situations when the hazard rate is not constant (but depends on time) we can sometimes use the Weibull distribution; this is also described.

The approach to survival time analysis using these two parametric models is compared with the non-parametric Kaplan–Meier method of estimating the survival curve.

3.1 THE EXPONENTIAL DISTRIBUTION

As indicated by equation (2.23) in section 2.13, there is a relationship between the hazard function, $h(t)$, and the survival function $S(t)$. In fact it is stated there that

$$h(t) = -\frac{d}{dt} [\log S(t)]. \qquad (3.1)$$

The right-hand side of equation (3.1) is the negative of the differential of the logarithm of $S(t)$ with respect to time t. Suppose we specify that the hazard does not change with time, t; i.e. we set

$$h(t) = \lambda, \tag{3.2}$$

where λ is a constant. Then, in this case, it turns out that the survival function, $S(t)$, has the form

$$S(t) = e^{-\lambda t}. \tag{3.3}$$

This is often written $S(t) = \exp(-\lambda t)$ and is termed the survival function of the exponential distribution. This constant hazard rate is a unique property of the exponential distribution and for this reason this distribution can play an important role in the description of survival data.

The shape of the exponential survival distribution of equation (3.3) is shown in Figure 3.1 for a particular value of the hazard rate $\lambda = 0.25$ per month. It is clear from this graph that only about 0.2 (20%) of the population remain alive at 6 months, less than 10% at 12 months, and there are very few survivors beyond 18 months. This is not very surprising since the hazard rate tells us that one-quarter of those alive at a given time will die in the following month.

For a value of the hazard rate $\lambda < 0.25$ the exponential survival function will lie above that of Figure 3.1 since the death rate is lower; for $\lambda > 0.25$ it will fall below since, in this case, the death rate is higher.

A constant value of the hazard rate implies that the probability of death remains constant as successive days go by. This idea extends to saying that the probability of death in any time interval depends only on the width of the interval. Thus the wider the time interval the greater the probability of death in that interval, but where the interval begins (and ends) has no influence on the death rate.

Example

Figure 3.2 shows the exponential survival function fitted to the survival time data

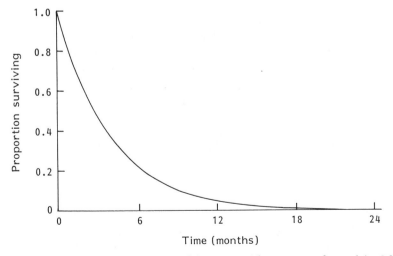

Figure 3.1 The exponential survival function with a constant hazard $\lambda = 0.25$

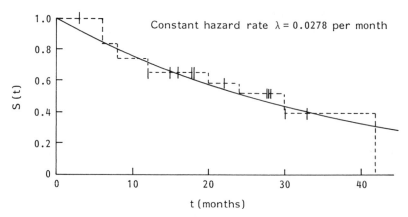

Figure 3.2 Exponential survival distribution fitted to the Dukes' C colorectal cancer data of McIllmurray and Turkie, 1987. Reproduced by permission of *Br. Med. J.* 294: 1260 and 295: 475.

of the 24 patients with Dukes' C colorectal cancer used to construct Figure 2.4. It is clear that the exponential survival function provides a close, but smoothed, summary of the Kaplan–Meier survival curve. Since there is a close fit of the exponential survival function to these data we can conclude that patients with this disease are therefore dying at an approximately constant rate. We can see that the risk of death does not appear to change with each succeeding month. It is worth highlighting that, in contrast to the Kaplan–Meier estimate of the survival curve, the exponential survival function extends beyond the time of death of the longest surviving patient, i.e. beyond $t = 42$ months.

3.2   ESTIMATING A CONSTANT HAZARD RATE

As we have already indicated in section 2.11, an overall estimate of the hazard rate, λ, is given by the number of deaths observed, d, divided by the total follow-up or exposure time. If t_i represents the individual survival times of the d patients who have died then their total follow-up is $f = \Sigma t_i$, and if T_j^+ represents the individual survival times of the $(n - d)$ patients still alive and who, therefore, have censored survival times, then their total follow-up is $F = \Sigma T_j^+$. Thus

$$\lambda = d/(f + F). \qquad (3.4)$$

Here $(f + F)$ can be thought of as the total follow-up time (or total period of observation), calculated from all patients in the study.

Example

If we were able to assume that the death rate, following the diagnosis of Dukes's C colorectal cancer, is constant in those patients studied by McIllmurray and Turkie (1987), then $d = 12$, $f = \Sigma t_i = 6 + 6 + 6 + 6 + 8 + 8 + 12 + 12 + 20 + 24 + 30 + 42 = 180$,

$F = \Sigma T_j^+ = 3 + 12 + 15 + 16 + 18 + 18 + 22 + 28 + 28 + 28 + 30 + 33 = 251$. This gives the total follow-up as $f + F = 180 + 251 = 431$ months; therefore from equation (3.4) $\lambda = 12/431 = 0.0278$. On an annual (12-month) basis the constant hazard rate is estimated to be $0.0278 \times 12 = 0.3336$ or 33%. This implies that approximately one-third of those patients alive at the beginning of a year die in that year.

If we had observed the times of death of all patients then there are no censored survival times. In this case $d = n$, the number of patients in the study, and we therefore observe a time to death t_i $(i = 1, 2, \ldots, n)$ for each patient. In this situation $\lambda = n/f = n/\Sigma t_i = 1/\bar{t}$, where $\bar{t}$ is the mean survival time. We would have this estimate if we had awaited the death of all 24 patients. In contrast, if no patients have yet died $(d = 0)$ the estimate of $\lambda = 0/F$ is zero, whatever the value of $F = \Sigma T_j^+$, the total (censored) survival time.

3.3   ASSESSING THE ASSUMPTION OF A CONSTANT HAZARD RATE

If we can assume a constant hazard rate $h(t) = \lambda$, i.e. one that does not change with time t, then, from equation (3.3) we obtain

$$\log[S(t)] = -\lambda t \tag{3.5}$$

or

$$-\log[S(t)] = \lambda t.$$

Further, if we then take the logarithms of each side of this latter equation we obtain

$$\log\{-\log[S(t)]\} = \log \lambda + \log t. \tag{3.6}$$

This is the form of an equation of a straight line $y = a + bx$, where $y = \log\{-\log[S(t)]\}$ is the left-hand side of equation (3.6). On the right-hand side of the equation, we have $a = \log \lambda$ as the intercept, $b = 1$ is the slope of the line and $x = \log t$.

Note that we have introduced $\log \{-\log[S(t)]\}$ when obtaining a CI for $S(t)$ by use of equation (2.14).

The straight-line form of equation (3.6) is shown in Figure 3.3 for the exponential survival function with $\lambda = 0.25$. When time $t = 1$, and hence $\log t = 0$, then the right-hand side of equation (3.6) is $\log \lambda$, which is the value on the vertical axis as indicated by the hatched lines in Figure 3.3. In this case $\log \lambda = \log 0.25 = -1.386$.

With a real data example, $\log \{-\log[S(t)]\}$ is plotted against $\log t$, where $S(t)$ is the Kaplan–Meier estimate of the survival function at each successive death time t. If this graph is approximately a straight line then we may assume that there is constant hazard rate. The intercept of such a graph for time $t = 1$ $(\log t = 0)$ provides an estimate of $\log \lambda$ and hence λ, the constant hazard rate. Systematic departures from a straight line indicate that it is not appropriate to assume λ is constant. In such circumstances the value of the hazard rate depends on t and therefore changes as time passes.

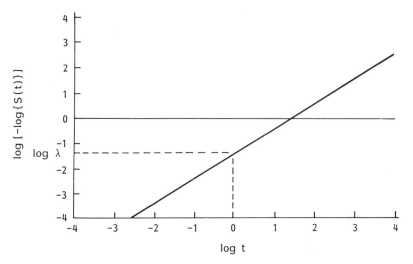

Figure 3.3 Graph of log{−log[S(t)]} against the logarithm of time, log t, for the exponential survival function with $\lambda = 0.25$ of Figure 3.1

Example

Table 3.1 summarises the calculations necessary for such a plot using the Kaplan–Meier estimates of S(t) from Table 2.2 for the data of McIllmurray and Turkie (1987). It is only possible to calculate the plot at time points when a death occurs and the value of S(t) changes. The final death at $t = 42$ months with $S(42) = 0.0000$ is omitted since the logarithm of zero is not defined.

There are six points here rather than the 12 which would have occurred if there were no tied observations. These six points are plotted in Figure 3.4. This graph indicates an approximate linear form and hence the assumption of a constant hazard rate seems reasonable for these patients.

Table 3.1 Calculations necessary for testing for a constant hazard rate using the data of McIllmurray and Turkie, 1987. Reproduced by permission of *Br. Med. J.* 294: 1260 and 295: 475.

Survival time t (months)	log t	Kaplan–Meier Estimate S(t)	log[S(t)]	log{−log[S(t)]}
6	1.79	0.8261	−0.1910	−1.66
8	2.08	0.7391	−0.3023	−1.20
12	2.48	0.6522	−0.4274	−0.85
20	3.00	0.5780	−0.5482	−0.60
24	3.18	0.5136	−0.6663	−0.41
30	3.40	0.3852	−0.9540	−0.05
42	3.74	0.0000	−	−

Drawing a straight line through the data points (by eye) and extending it downwards to cut the log (time) axis at zero gives the intercept log $\lambda = -3.24$ as indicated in Figure 3.4. From this we have $\lambda = \exp(-3.24) = 0.0392 \approx 0.04$.

This contrasts somewhat with the estimator of $\lambda = 0.0278$ (≈ 0.03) given earlier but the discrepancy is likely to be caused by drawing the line by eye, the intercept is far removed from the data points, and there is presence of both a large proportion of censored observations (50%) and tied observations in these data.

The expression given in equation (3.4) should always be preferred to calculate λ as it makes full use of the censored survival times and the tied observations. Nevertheless, the graph gives an indication that the use of equation (3.4) for the calculation of the hazard rate is appropriate.

As we have already noted from equation (3.6) the slope of the fitted line, the multiplier of log t, is unity, and so if the exponential distribution is appropriate then the slope, b, of Figure 3.4 should be approximately unity.

In fact, we can estimate b from the graph by calculating the change in y divided by the corresponding change in x. To do this we take any two values for x (say)

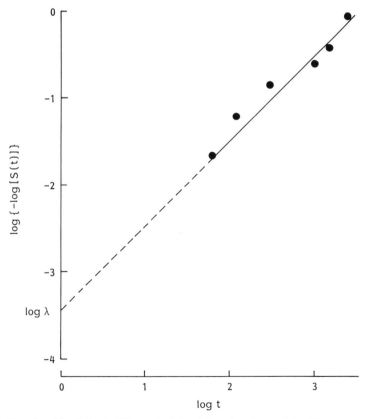

Figure 3.4 Graph of log{−log[s(t)]} against log t for the data of McIllmurray and Turkie, 1987. Reproduced by permission of *Br. Med. J.* 294: 1260 and 295: 475.

$x_1 = \log t_1 = 1$ and $x_2 = \log t_2 = 3$ for convenience, with corresponding values $y_1 = -2.46$ and $y_2 = -0.52$. These give

$$b = \frac{y_2 - y_1}{x_2 - x_1} = \frac{-0.52 - (-2.46)}{3 - 1} = \frac{1.94}{2} = 0.97$$

which is close to unity. This gives further support for the use of the exponential distribution in describing these data as b is close to unity.

3.4   CONFIDENCE INTERVALS FOR THE HAZARD RATE

It can be shown that if the number of events (deaths) is large, then an approximate 95% CI can be obtained for λ in the usual way, from

$$\lambda - 1.96 SE(\lambda) \quad \text{to} \quad \lambda + 1.96 SE(\lambda). \tag{3.7}$$

The expression for $SE(\lambda)$ depends on whether or not censored observations are present. If not, i.e. the critical event is observed in all n subjects, then an estimate of the $SE(\lambda)$ is given by

$$SE(\lambda) = \lambda/\sqrt{n}. \tag{3.8}$$

In the presence of censoring a corresponding estimate of the SE is

$$SE(\lambda) = \lambda/\sqrt{(d-1)} \tag{3.9}$$

where d is the number of events observed.

Example

Applying equation (3.9) to the Dukes' C colorectal cancer data with $d = 12$, $\lambda = 0.0278$ (but remembering that the number of deaths here is quite small) gives $SE(\lambda) = 0.0278/\sqrt{11} = 0.008395$. A 95% CI for λ is therefore $0.0278 - 1.96 \times 0.008395$ to $0.0278 + 1.96 \times 0.008395$ or 0.0113 to 0.0442 per month. On an annual basis this is 14% to 53%, which is extremely wide, as one might expect from such a small study.
   An alternative method of calculating a 95% CI is to use the expression

$$\log \lambda - 1.96 SE (\log \lambda) \quad \text{to} \quad \log \lambda + 1.96 SE (\log \lambda) \tag{3.10}$$

since $\log \lambda$ often follows more closely a Normal distribution than does λ itself. In this case

$$SE(\log \lambda) = 1/\sqrt{d}. \tag{3.11}$$

Substituting $\lambda = 0.0278$ in equation (3.10) gives $\log \lambda = -3.5827$, $SE(\log \lambda) = 1/\sqrt{12} = 0.2887$ and the 95% CI for $\log \lambda$ as $-3.5827 - 1.96 \times 0.2887$ to $-3.5827 + 1.96 \times 0.2887$ or -4.1485 to -3.0169. If we exponentiate both limits of this interval we obtain $\exp(-4.1485) = 0.0158$ to $\exp(-3.0169) = 0.0490$ for the 95% CI for λ. These are very similar to those obtained previously but the CI is no longer symmetric about $\lambda = 0.0278$. It is preferable, however, always to use this latter approach as equation (3.7) can lead, for example, to negative values of the lower confidence limit.

3.5 THE WEIBULL DISTRIBUTION

The exponential distribution is a useful form of the survival distribution when the hazard rate, λ, is constant and does not depend on time. Thus, as time progresses for a particular individual, the probability of death in successive time intervals remains unchanged. There are, however, circumstances in which we know that this will not be the case. For example, following major surgery, death is more likely to occur in the immediate postoperative period in many situations but then may return to an approximately constant (and lower) level thereafter. In other words, the operative procedure itself brings a risk of death over and above that of the disease itself. There are other situations in which the (instantaneous) hazard could be increasing or decreasing with time. For example, a smoker ceasing to smoke may induce a decreasing mortality hazard (at least in the short term) compared to his hazard had he continued to smoke. It is also well known that the risk of death to a newborn infant is high in the first few days of life; thereafter it rapidly decreases and remains low and approximately constant, until much later in life, when it begins to increase again.

One way of making the hazard depend on time is to modify the exponential survival function of equation (3.3) in a simple way, as follows:

$$S(t) = \exp[-(\lambda t)^\kappa] \tag{3.12}$$

where κ is a constant whose value is greater than zero. This is known as the Weibull distribution. In the particular case of $\kappa = 1$ equation (3.12) becomes equation (3.3), and we have the exponential distribution again.

Equation (3.12) can be written as $\log[S(t)] = -(\lambda t)^\kappa$, which can be compared with equation (3.5). The hazard function is obtained from this expression by differentiating with respect to t (see equation (3.1)), to give

$$h(t) = \kappa\lambda(\lambda t)^{\kappa-1}. \tag{3.13}$$

This is known as the hazard function for the Weibull distribution and clearly depends on time, since t is included on the right-hand side of the expression.

This hazard function looks somewhat complicated but if we set $\kappa = 1$ in equation (3.13) then $h(t) = 1 \times \lambda(\lambda t)^{1-1} = \lambda(\lambda t)^0 = \lambda$. This is then the constant hazard of the exponential survival distribution that we had before.

Equation (3.13) gives a hazard rate which changes with time and whose shape depends on the value of κ. Some of these shapes are illustrated in Figure 3.5, with a value of $\lambda = 1$ used for simplicity. For example, with $\kappa = 0.5$, $h(t) = 0.5 \times 1 (t)^{0.5-1} = 0.5/\sqrt{t}$, and the hazard rate is at first very high indeed, then rapidly falls and is almost zero beyond $t = 3$. If $\kappa = 1$ then the hazard rate is the constant value of the exponential situation already referred to. For $\kappa = 2$, $h(t) = 2\lambda(\lambda t) = 2\lambda^2 t$ and the hazard rate increases with t in a linear way with slope

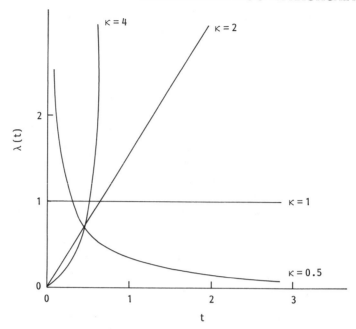

Figure 3.5   Hazard functions of the Weibull distribution with $\lambda = 1$ and varying values of κ

$2\lambda^2$. For $\kappa = 4$, $h(t) = 4\lambda^4 t^3$ and this hazard rate increases very steeply indeed from zero at time $t = 0$.

Such a range of shapes for the possible hazard function makes the Weibull distribution a good choice to describe a variety of survival time problems.

3.6   GRAPHICAL METHODS

A graphical test for suitability of the Weibull distribution to describe the data can be derived in a similar way to that for the exponential distribution. Thus taking logarithms, changing signs and taking logarithms again of equation (3.12), we have

$$\log\{-\log[S(t)]\} = \kappa \log \lambda + \kappa \log t. \qquad (3.14)$$

This expression reduces to equation (3.6) in the situation when $\kappa = 1$. The right-hand side of (3.14) is linear in $\log t$ and has intercept $a = \kappa \log \lambda$ and slope $b = \kappa$.

Hence a plot of $\log\{-\log[S(t)]\}$ against $\log t$ with a particular data set provides a graphical test of the Weibull distribution. If the resulting plot is indeed approximately a straight line with a slope not equal to unity, then this indicates that a Weibull distribution may describe the data sufficiently well.

Example

We use the data of McIllmurray and Turkie (1987) plotted in Figure 3.4 for illustration. As noted earlier the plot is approximately linear and we have calculated the slope $b = 0.97$. This provides us with our estimate of $\kappa = b = 0.97$. The intercept at $t = 1$ gives $a = \kappa \log \lambda = -3.24$ and therefore $\log \lambda = -3.24/\kappa = -3.24/0.97 = -3.340$. Finally $\lambda = \exp(-3.340) = 0.0354$. This estimate differs from the graphical estimate of the hazard rate for the exponential distribution given earlier.

3.7 ESTIMATING λ AND κ

To obtain the maximum likelihood estimates of λ and κ using the full information available rather than that provided by the graphical method of Figure 3.4, it is necessary to solve quite complicated equations. These equations are

$$W(\kappa) = \frac{\sum t_i^\kappa \log t_i + \sum T_j^{+\kappa} \log T_j^+}{\sum t_i^\kappa + \sum T_j^{+\kappa}} - \frac{\sum \log t_i}{d} - \frac{1}{\kappa} = 0 \tag{3.15}$$

and

$$\lambda = [d/(\sum t_i^\kappa + \sum T_j^{+\kappa})]^{1/\kappa}. \tag{3.16}$$

To solve equation (3.15) for κ involves finding a particular κ which makes $W(\kappa) = 0$. Once κ is obtained, λ is calculated using equation (3.16). One method of solving equation (3.15) is by 'trial and error'. For example, we can obtain an estimate of $\kappa = \kappa_G$ from the graphical method just described. We then substitute κ_G in equation (3.15) to obtain $W(\kappa_G)$. If this is zero then our graphical estimate itself is indeed the solution to the equation. More usually $W(\kappa_G) \neq 0$ and we need to choose a second value of κ, perhaps a little smaller (or larger) than κ_G and calculate $W(\kappa)$ again. If this is nearer to zero than $W(\kappa_G)$, then we are moving in the direction of the solution. The same process is repeated with differing values for κ until $W(\kappa) = 0$ is obtained. The corresponding value of κ is then the maximum likelihood solution, κ_{ML}, of equation (3.15). Substituting κ_{ML} in equation (3.16) gives the maximum likelihood estimate of λ, or λ_{ML}.

Example

From the graphical approach of section 3.6, we have $\kappa = 0.97$ for the data of McIllmurray and Turkie (1987). Details of the calculation of $W(0.97) = -0.4465$, are given in Table 3.2. Substituting the appropriate column totals in equation (3.15) gives

$$W(0.97) = \frac{491.7489 + 715.8394}{166.5359 + 228.4675} - \frac{29.6730}{12} - \frac{1}{0.97}$$

$$= 3.0572 - 2.4728 - 1.0309$$

$$= -0.4465.$$

This is clearly not equal to zero and so a different value for κ is required. Table 3.3 gives the value of $W(\kappa)$ for differing values of κ and shows that when $\kappa = 1.4294$, $W(\kappa) = 0$. We then use $\kappa_{ML} = 1.4294$ in equation (3.16) to obtain $\lambda_{ML} = 0.0319$. The

Table 3.2 Summary of calculations to obtain $W(\kappa)$ as a step to obtaining the maximum likelihood estimate of κ for a Weibull distribution

t_i	t_i^κ	$\log t_i$	$t_i^\kappa \log t_i$	T_i^+	$T_i^{+\kappa}$	$\log T_i^+$	$T_i^{+\kappa} \log T_i^+$
6	5.6860	1.7918	10.1879	3	2.9027	1.0986	3.1890
6	5.6860	1.7918	10.1879	12	11.1380	2.4849	27.6768
6	5.6860	1.7918	10.1879	15	13.8296	2.7081	37.4512
6	5.6860	1.7918	10.1879	16	14.7230	2.7726	40.8208
8	7.5162	2.0794	15.6295	18	16.5050	2.8904	47.7055
8	7.5162	2.0794	15.6295	18	16.5050	2.8904	47.7055
12	11.1380	2.4849	27.6768	22	20.0516	3.0910	61.9805
12	11.1380	2.4849	27.6768	28	25.3363	3.3322	84.4258
20	18.2810	2.9957	54.7649	28	25.3363	3.3322	84.4258
24	21.8175	3.1781	69.3372	28	25.3363	3.3322	84.4258
32	28.8400	3.4657	99.9519	30	27.0899	3.4012	92.1381
42	37.5450	3.7377	140.3307	33	29.7138	3.4965	103.8946
Total	166.5359	29.6730	491.7489		228.4675		715.8394

Table 3.3 Summary of the iterative calculations necessary to estimate λ of the Weibull distribution

κ	$W(\kappa)$	λ
0.97	−0.4465	0.0273
1	−0.4070	0.0277
1.2	−0.1871	0.0301
1.4	−0.0211	0.0317
1.4294	0.0000	0.0319
1.5	0.0478	0.0323

final Weibull fit to the Kaplan–Meier survival curve is shown in Figure 3.6. This describes the data reasonably well but differs from the exponential fit of Figure 3.2 in that there is a small 'shoulder' in the early part of the curve. A formal test of whether there is a significant improvement in fit by the (two-parameter, λ and κ) Weibull distribution over the (one-parameter, λ) exponential distribution can be made by means of a likelihood ratio (LR) test introduced in section 1.6. We do not describe this test here.

3.8   PARAMETRIC VERSUS NON-PARAMETRIC METHODS

The exponential distribution is fully described once we know the value of the parameter λ. Similarly, once we know the two parameters λ and κ, we can then describe the Weibull distribution. In practice, we estimate these parameters from the data provided. In fact, once the estimates of these parameters are obtained it is no longer strictly essential to retain the individual survival times. However, it is

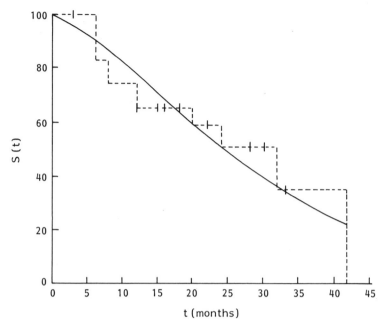

Figure 3.6 The fitted Weibull distribution, with $\lambda_{ML} = 0.0319$, $\kappa_{ML} = 1.4294$, for the data of McIllmurray and Turkie, 1987. Reproduced by permission of *Br. Med. J.* 294: 1260 and 295: 475.

usually valuable to present both the (smooth) exponential or Weibull curve with the corresponding Kaplan–Meier (non-parametric) estimate superimposed.

In contrast, the non-parametric Kaplan–Meier estimate of the survival curve retains the individual patient data when presented. Indeed, it is more usual to use the Kaplan–Meier description of the data and not to pursue an underlying distributional form. This contrasts quite markedly to other branches of statistical methods where there are considerable advantages in being able to assume that the data (or some transformation of it) have a Normal distribution form.

In general, it is now not very common to use a parametric distribution, for example the Weibull, to describe the data, as these may require some investigation to establish their use, and raise difficulties in the estimation of the parameters. Such techniques were necessary, however, prior to the time that the Cox proportional hazards model of chapter 6 was proposed (see section 11.4 for an example of a Cox model and a Weibull model fitted to the same data). Then, it was useful to obtain a parametric model of the data. This could then be used with standard regression techniques to investigate prognostic variables, for example.

3.9 TECHNICAL DETAILS

Rather than denote death times by t_i and censored times by T_j^+, it is often convenient to incorporate these two types of time into one. To do this we think of each patient, i, having an observed survival time t_i which is a death time if an associated variable $\delta_i = 1$ and is censored if $\delta_i = 0$. Thus we can write, for the ith patient, the pair (t_i, δ_i) to describe the survival time and status. This device is often used in statistical packages; thus one (column) variable denotes the survival time and the second (column) the survival status (dead = 1, alive = 0).

If we can assume a constant hazard, then for a patient who has died $\delta_i = 1$ and the probability of death at t_i is (since the distribution of survival times is exponential) $\lambda e^{-\lambda t_i}$. If the patient has not died $\delta_i = 0$ then all we can calculate is the probability of survival beyond t_i which is $e^{-\lambda t_i}$. In general, the probability of death at time t_i for patient i, can be written

$$l_i(\lambda) = (\lambda e^{-\lambda t_i})^{\delta_i}(e^{-\lambda t_i})^{1 - \delta_i}$$
$$= \lambda^{\delta_i} e^{-\lambda t_i}. \tag{3.17}$$

Equation (3.17) is often termed the likelihood for patient i from which $L_i(\lambda) = \log l_i(\lambda) = \delta_i \log \lambda - \lambda t$. If we differentiate $L_i(\delta)$ with respect to λ then we obtain

$$\frac{dL_i(\lambda)}{d\lambda} = [\delta_i/\lambda - t_i]. \tag{3.18}$$

The expression

$$U_i(\lambda) = \delta_i/\lambda - t_i \tag{3.19}$$

is termed the efficient score statistic.

If we calculate U_i for all n patients and set $\Sigma U_i(\lambda) = 0$ then this leads to $\lambda = \Sigma \delta_i/\Sigma t_i$. This is the form of equation (3.4) with $\Sigma \delta_i$ replaced by the total number of observed deaths (d) and Σt_i replaced by the sum of all the survival times $(f + F)$ whether censored or not. As a consequence, the estimate (3.4) is known as the maximum likelihood estimate of λ.

4 | Comparison of Two Survival Curves

Summary

This chapter describes the logrank test to compare two Kaplan–Meier survival curves. The hazard ratio (HR) is introduced as a useful single measure for summarising the differences between two survival curves. Methods of calculation of confidence intervals for the HR are described. The logrank test is extended to a stratified analysis in which, for example, the influence of a prognostic variable is taken into account. Other tests, which may be more appropriate than the logrank test in some situations, are also given.

4.1 INTRODUCTION

In chapter 2, we described how the Kaplan–Meier estimate of a single survival curve is obtained. However, in many applications, there will often be several survival curves to compare. Thus we may wish to compare the survival experiences of patients who receive different treatments for their disease, or compare the discontinuation rates in women using one of two types of intrauterine device for fertility control. In such circumstances, for two groups we require a procedure similar to that of the Student's t-test for normally distributed data. Before we describe the methods available to compare two survival curves, we note that it is inappropriate and usually very misleading to compare survival curves at a particular point of the curve, for example, making comparisons of 1-year survival rates. The reason for this is that each *individual point* on the curve is not in itself a good estimate of the true underlying survival. Thus comparing two such estimates (one from each of the two curves) leads to an unreliable comparison of the survival experience of the two groups. Further, it makes very poor use of all the data available by concentrating on particular points of each curve and ignoring the remainder of the survival experience.

4.2   THE LOGRANK TEST

We have given in chapter 2 several examples of the Kaplan–Meier survival curves. There are many situations, particularly in the context of randomised trials and epidemiological studies, in which we may wish to compare two or more such curves. The logrank test, also referred to as the Mantel–Cox test, is the most widely used method of comparing two survival curves and can easily be extended to comparisons of three or more curves.

Example from the literature

The Kaplan–Meier estimates of the survival curves for patients with chronic heart failure receiving treatment with either placebo or milrinone reported by Packer *et al.* (1991) are illustrated in Figure 4.1. The numbers of patients at risk, at 3-monthly intervals, are shown at the bottom of the figure.

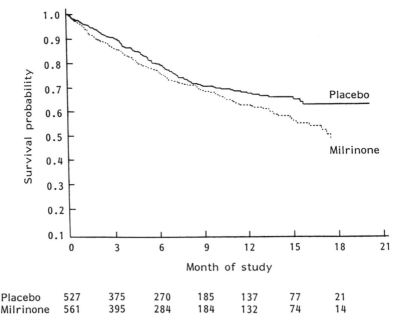

Placebo	527	375	270	185	137	77	21
Milrinone	561	395	284	184	132	74	14

Figure 4.1 Kaplan–Meier analysis showing survival in patients with chronic heart failure treated with milrinone or placebo (From Packer *et al.*, 1991. Reprinted by permission of *The New England Journal of Medicine* 325: 1468–75. © 1991 Massachusetts Medical Society)

The authors report the result of a logrank test of significance for the comparison of these two groups and from this they conclude that there is a greater death rate amongst patients receiving milrinone. They state: 'Mortality was 28% higher in the milrinone group than in the placebo group (p = 0.038)'.

To illustrate the logrank test, Table 4.1 shows the survival times of 30 patients recruited to a randomised trial of the addition of a radiosensitiser to radiotherapy (New therapy, B) versus radiotherapy alone (Control, A) in patients with cervical cancer. Of these 30 patients, 16 received A and 14 received B. These data are a subset of those obtained from 183 patients entered into a randomised Phase III trial conducted by the MRC Working Party on Advanced Carcinoma of the Cervix (1993). We refer to the treatments as A and B for ease and because we do not intend to draw conclusions on the relative effect of the two treatments in such a small subset of patients.

Now if the two treatments are of equal efficacy, i.e. the addition of the radiosensitiser to radiotherapy has no effect, then the corresponding survival curves should only differ because of chance variation. Thus, under the assumption of no difference between the two treatments, we anticipate that the two patient groups will have a similar survival experience. This should be the case, at least approximately, if allocation to treatment is random and the groups are of sufficient size.

Now, we can check for balance of *known* factors which are likely to influence prognosis (prognostic factors). For example, the age of the patient may be an

Table 4.1 Survival by treatment group of 30 patients recruited to a cervical cancer trial. (Based on data from MRC Working Party on Advanced Carcinoma of the Cervix, 1993. Reproduced by permission of *Radiotherapy Oncology* 26: 93–103.)

Control A			New therapy B		
Patient number	Survival time	Survival status	Patient number	Survival time	Survival status
2	1037	DEAD	1	1476+	ALIVE
4	1429	DEAD	3	827	DEAD
5	680	DEAD	7	519+	ALIVE
6	291	DEAD	8	1100+	ALIVE
9	1577+	ALIVE	10	1307	DEAD
11	90	DEAD	12	1360+	ALIVE
14	1090+	ALIVE	13	919+	ALIVE
15	142	DEAD	16	373	DEAD
17	1297	DEAD	18	563+	ALIVE
19	1113+	ALIVE	21	978+	ALIVE
20	1153	DEAD	22	650+	ALIVE
23	150	DEAD	25	362	DEAD
24	837	DEAD	27	383+	ALIVE
26	890+	ALIVE	28	272	DEAD
29	269	DEAD			
30	468+	ALIVE			

important determinant of prognosis and we can check that the two groups have similar age distributions. However, we cannot check balance for *unknown* prognostic factors. Thus, any observed differences between the two curves and which we would like to ascribe to differences between treatments may be explained by chance differences due to a maldistribution of unknown prognostic factors.

When patients have been allocated randomly to the two treatments, the p-value obtained from the significance test allows us to make statements about how likely it is that an observed difference between treatments is due to an imbalance in (known and unknown) prognostic factors. In a non-randomised study the p-value, although still a useful tool in the test of the null hypothesis of 'no difference' between treatments, does not have the same interpretation.

For the trial in patients with cervical cancer, treatment was indeed allocated at random. However, the patient groups selected for purposes of illustration are very small, with a total of only 30 patients, so imbalances of known and unknown prognostic variables in the two groups are very likely.

The Kaplan–Meier survival curves for the groups A and B of Table 4.1 are shown in Figure 4.2 and appear to be quite different. However, how different do they have

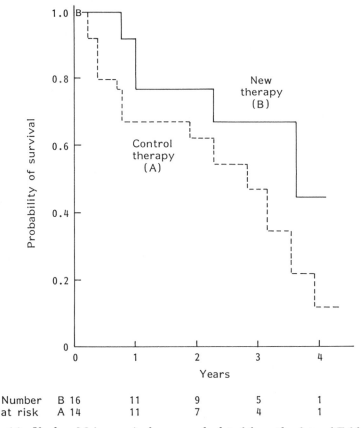

| Number | B 16 | 11 | 9 | 5 | 1 |
| at risk | A 14 | 11 | 7 | 4 | 1 |

Figure 4.2 Kaplan–Meier survival curves calculated from the data of Table 4.1

to appear to be before we can *reliably* attribute this difference to a treatment effect? How can we be sure that the difference is not due to an imbalance in known and unknown prognostic factors? How different must they be in order to reject the (null) hypothesis of 'no treatment difference'?

To make a formal comparison of these two survival curves we first rank the survival times of all 30 patients, using the convention already stated in chapter 2, that if a 'death' and a 'censored' observation have the same numerical value we will allocate the censored time a higher rank. This ranking has been done in two stages: first the survival times are ranked within each treatment group as in Table 4.2 and then, for all data combined, irrespective of treatment, in the first two columns of Table 4.3. The two columns are separated, one for each treatment, only for the sake of clarity. Note that there is a tendency for those on treatment B to have a higher ranking and thus experiencing later deaths than those receiving A, as would be expected from Figure 4.2.

Before going into full details of how the logrank test is calculated we illustrate the approach by examining the 2×2 table corresponding to the first death of Table 4.3 which occurred on day 90 to a patient receiving treatment A. This table is reproduced in Table 4.4 together with the notation we shall use to describe the logrank test procedure.

From Table 4.2 (and Table 4.3) we see for this patient receiving treatment A who died on day 90 following randomisation that just before her death there were 30 patients alive: 16 on treatment A and 14 on treatment B. If we were told of the occurrence of one death at this stage (without knowledge of the particular

Table 4.2 Ranked within-treatment survival times of 30 patients recruited to a cervical cancer trial

Control A			New therapy B		
Patient number	Survival time (days)	Survival status	Patient number	Survival time (days)	Survival status
11	90	DEAD	28	272	DEAD
15	142	DEAD	25	362	DEAD
23	150	DEAD	16	373	DEAD
29	269	DEAD	27	383+	ALIVE
6	291	DEAD	7	519+	ALIVE
30	468+	ALIVE	18	563+	ALIVE
5	680	DEAD	22	650+	ALIVE
24	837	DEAD	3	827	DEAD
26	890+	ALIVE	13	919+	ALIVE
2	1037	DEAD	21	978+	ALIVE
14	1090+	ALIVE	8	1100+	ALIVE
19	1113+	ALIVE	10	1307	DEAD
20	1153	DEAD	12	1360+	ALIVE
17	1297	DEAD	1	1476+	ALIVE
4	1429	DEAD			
9	1577+	ALIVE			

Table 4.3 Ranked survival times of 30 patients with cervical cancer by treatment group

Patient number	Rank	Survival (days) A	B		Dead	Alive	Total	E_{At}	E_{Bt}	V_t
11	1	90		A	1	15	16			
				B	0	14	14			
					1	29	30	0.533333	0.466667	0.248889
15	2	142		A	1	14	15			
				B	0	14	14			
					1	28	29	0.517241	0.482759	0.249703
23	3	150		A	1	13	14			
				B	0	14	14			
					1	27	28	0.500000	0.500000	0.250000
29	4	269		A	1	12	13			
				B	0	14	14			
					1	26	27	0.481481	0.518519	0.249657
28	5		272	A	0	12	12			
				B	1	13	14			
					1	25	26	0.461538	0.538462	0.248521
22	6	291		A	1	11	12			
				B	0	13	13			
					1	24	25	0.480000	0.520000	0.249600
6	7		362	A	0	11	11			
				B	1	12	13			
					1	23	24	0.458333	0.541667	0.248264
25	8		373	A	0	11	11			
				B	1	11	12			
					1	22	23	0.478261	0.521739	0.249527
27	9		383+							
30	10	468+								
7	11		519+							
18	12		563+							
22	13		650+							
5	14	680		A	1	9	10			
				B	0	7	7			
					1	16	17	0.588235	0.411765	0.242215
3	15		827	A	0	9	9			
				B	1	6	7			
					1	15	16	0.562500	0.437500	0.246094

Table 4.3 (*continued*)

Patient number	Rank	Survival (days) A	B		Dead	Alive	Total	E_{At}	E_{Bt}	V_t
24	16	837		A	1	8	9			
				B	0	6	6			
					1	14	15	0.600000	0.400000	0.240000
26	17	890+								
13	18		919+							
21	19		978+							
2	20	1037		A	1	6	7			
				B	0	4	4			
					1	10	11	0.636364	0.363636	0.231405
14	21	1090+								
8	22		1100+							
19	23	1113+								
20	24	1153		A	1	3	4			
				B	0	3	3			
					1	6	7	0.571429	0.428571	0.244898
17	25	1297		A	1	2	3			
				B	0	3	3			
					1	5	6	0.500000	0.500000	0.250000
10	26		1307	A	0	2	2			
				B	1	2	3			
					1	4	5	0.400000	0.600000	0.240000
12	27		1360+							
4	28	1429		A	1	1	2			
				B	0	1	1			
					1	2	3	0.666667	0.333333	0.222222
1	29		1476+							
9	30	1577+								
		Total		$O_A = 11$		$O_B = 5$		$E_A = 8.435382$	$E_B = 7.564618$	$V = 3.910995$

treatment group in which the death occurred) then, under the null hypothesis of no difference in the treatments, we can calculate the odds of this death for A and B. This will take account of the number of patients known to be receiving A (m_{90}) and B (n_{90}). Thus for the one death at $t = 90$ days, we calculate the odds as m_{90} to n_{90} or $16 : 14$ and so the expected number of deaths on treatment A is $E_{A,90} = 16/(16 + 14) = 0.533333$ and the expected number of deaths on treatment B is $E_{B,90} = 14/(16 + 14) = 0.466667$. These are given in the top panel of Table 4.4. We discuss the definition and use of V_t in section 4.5.

This calculation is equivalent to calculating the expected values in a standard

Table 4.4 Comparison of observed and expected deaths following the first death at 90 days and the general notation used at time t

Time t = 90 Treatment	Dead	Alive	Total	$E_{A,90}$	$E_{B,90}$	V_{90}
A	1	15	16			
B	0	14	14			
Total	1	29	30	0.533333	0.466667	0.248889

Time t Treatment	Dead	Alive	Total	E_{At}	E_{Bt}	V_t
A	a_t	c_t	m_t			
B	b_t	d_t	n_t			
Total	r_t	s_t	N_t	$\dfrac{r_t m_t}{N_t}$	$\dfrac{r_t n_t}{N_t}$	$\dfrac{m_t n_t r_t s_t}{N_t^2(N_t - 1)}$

2×2 contingency table at t = 90, with $r_{90} = 1$, $m_{90} = 16$ and $N_{90} = 30$, as is indicated in the lower panel of Table 4.4. We then compare the observed number of deaths, $a_t = 1$ and $b_t = 0$, with these expected values. It is a common convention to call $a_t = O_{At}$ and $b_t = O_{Bt}$, respectively. Thus, there are more deaths under A (here $O_{A,90} = 1$ death) than expected (0.533333) but fewer under B (here $O_{B,90} = 0$ deaths) than expected (0.466667). If there is only one death at the time, then the expected number of deaths can also be interpreted as the probability of the death occurring in each treatment group.

This basic calculation is then repeated at each death time. For the second death at t = 142, we have $O_{A,142} = 1$ and $O_{B,142} = 0$. However, as with the Kaplan–Meier estimate, we do not carry forward the patient receiving treatment A who died at t = 90, so the odds of death at t = 142 are divided in the ratio 15:14 rather than the 16:14 at t = 90. This gives $E_{A,142} = 15/(15 + 14) = 0.517241$ and $E_{B,142} = 14/(15 + 14) = 0.482759$.

In general the expected number of deaths for A and B at death time t are calculated by

$$E_{At} = r_t m_t / N_t$$
$$E_{Bt} = r_t n_t / N_t \tag{4.1}$$

as indicated in Table 4.4. This takes into account the situation of tied observations when two or more deaths occur at a particular time t.

The process of calculating the expected values continues for every successive 2×2 table. There is one formed for each distinct time of death, with the margins of the table for either A or B or both decreasing death by death. In addition, if censored observations occur between death times then the respective marginal totals for A (m_t) and/or B (n_t) are reduced and the 2×2 table is formed at the next death with these reduced margins. This process is illustrated by considering the death on treatment B at 373 days: just before this death there are 23 patients still at risk. This death is followed by five censored observations: 468^+ for treatment A, and 383^+, 519^+, 563^+ and 650^+ for treatment B (see Table 4.4). As a consequence, the next 2×2 table is formed at $t = 680$ and is made up from the 17 patients still at risk: 10 on treatment A and 7 on treatment B.

Once these calculations are completed, i.e. all deaths have been included, the observed and expected deaths are summed, to give

$$O_A = \Sigma \, O_{At}, \qquad E_A = \Sigma \, E_{At}$$
$$O_B = \Sigma \, O_{Bt}, \qquad E_B = \Sigma \, E_{Bt}. \tag{4.2}$$

Finally the logrank statistic is calculated as

$$\chi^2_{\text{Logrank}} = \frac{(O_A - E_A)^2}{E_A} + \frac{(O_B - E_B)^2}{E_B}. \tag{4.3}$$

This is a format which is similar to that for the standard χ^2 test of equation (1.11) (see, for example, Campbell and Machin, 1993, p. 80, for a more complete description).

From Table 4.1 we obtain $O_A = 11$, $E_A = 8.435382$, $O_B = 5$ and $E_B = 7.564618$. These give $(O_A - E_A) = 2.564618$ indicating more deaths than expected on treatment A, and $(O_B - E_B) = -2.564618$ or fewer deaths than expected on treatment B. Finally

$$\chi^2_{\text{Logrank}} = (2.564618)^2/8.435382 + (-2.564618)^2/7.564618$$
$$= 1.649201.$$

In general for G treatment groups the χ^2_{Logrank} is compared with the χ^2 distribution with $G - 1$ degrees of freedom. Thus for two treatment groups χ^2_{Logrank} is compared with the χ^2 distribution with degrees of freedom $df = 2 - 1 = 1$. Using the first row of Table T3 we obtain an approximate p-value of 0.2. This is not statistically significant at the 0.05 (5%) level. In this situation, as indicated in section 1.6, an exact p-value is obtained by referring $z = \sqrt{\chi^2_{\text{Logrank}}} = \sqrt{1.649201} \approx 1.28$ to Table T1, which gives a p-value = 0.2005. Thus this result, although not conventionally statistically significant at the 5% level, suggests that treatment B may be better than treatment A. However, this is certainly not conclusive evidence. A larger study is required to reliably confirm or refute this result. We discuss in section 4.4 how important it is to quote appropriate CIs to reflect the uncertainty in such situations.

It is useful to note, since E_A and E_B are the sums of a large number of small quantities, that it is practice to calculate the individual components, E_{At} and E_{Bt}, to sufficient (many) decimal places just as for the calculations of the Kaplan–Meier estimate of the survival curves. Since $E_A + E_B$ must also equal the total number of deaths $O_A + O_B$, it is not strictly necessary to calculate the individual components of E_B since

$$E_B = (O_A + O_B) - E_A.$$

It is, however, a useful check on the arithmetic if E_B is calculated from the sum of the individual E_{Bt} rather than merely from this difference.

It is also important to note that in a study in which all the patients have died and, therefore, there is 100% mortality in both (all) groups, provided we have their survival times recorded, then the corresponding E can exceed O, the total number of patients (here also deaths), in a single group. This is because the expectations, E, are calculated using the assumption that the death rates are common in the two (or more) groups and therefore the group with the largest summed survival time should 'expect' more deaths, in which case E will be greater than O. On the other hand, the treatment in which the patients die more quickly will have an E less than the corresponding O.

Example from the literature

Cheingsong-Popov *et al.* (1991) compared the time to progression to Stage IV disease in patients with AIDS whose gag (p24) antibody levels are 1600 or more with those with fewer antibodies.

Their results are summarised in Figure 4.3, which suggests that the disease of patients with the fewer gag (p24) antibodies may progress more quickly. They quote a significance test with p-value = 0.0008, which would correspond to a χ^2_{Logrank} with one degree of freedom (df = 1) of approximately 7.1.

This example illustrates the use of the survival techniques for a between-group comparison where the group is defined by a characteristic of the individuals under study and not by the investigator as, for example, would be the case of the treatment given to a patient in a clinical trial.

Example from the literature

The World Health Organization (WHO, 1988) conducted an international multicentre randomised trial of two, once-monthly injectable contraceptives,

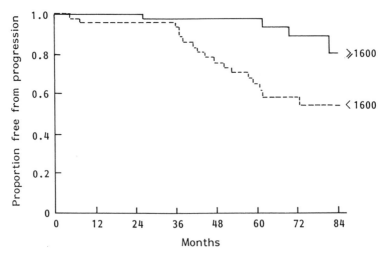

Figure 4.3 Kaplan–Meier survival analysis for time to progression to stage IV disease by gag (p24) antibody levels (From Cheingsong-Popov *et al.*, 1991, reproduced by permission of *Br. Med. J.* 302, 23–26. (Published by BMJ Publishing Group))

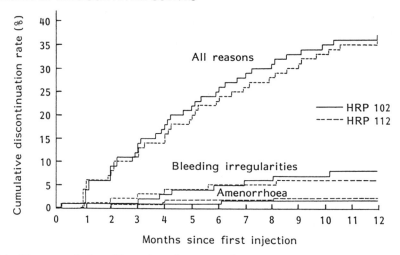

Figure 4.4 The cumulative discontinuation rates in women using two, once-monthly, injectable contraceptives for amenorrhoea, bleeding irregularities and all reasons including women lost to follow-up (From World Health Organization Task Force on Long-acting Systemic Agents for Fertility Regulation, 1988, with permission)

HRP102 and HRP112, in 2328 women. Figure 4.4 shows the cumulative method discontinuation rates for all reasons by type of injectable contraceptive. In this situation losses to follow-up are not censored but are regarded as events (failure to continue with the method) since it is presumed that women who do not return to the clinic for the next injection are not satisfied with the method. They are not therefore 'true' losses to follow-up in this context. The trial only continues for 1 year, so that all subjects have this as the maximum observation time. The time of 1 year will provide a censored observation for all those women who continue method use up to this time. From these data there is little evidence of a difference between the discontinuation rates with either contraceptive method.

Of particular interest in this trial was the comparison of bleeding-related, including amenorrhoea, discontinuation rates. These were 6.3% and 7.5% at 1 year for HRP112 and HRP102, respectively. A formal logrank test of this difference in discontinuation rates gave $\chi^2_{Logrank} = 0.77$, df = 1, p-value = 0.38.

We note that equation (4.3) can be written as

$$\chi^2_{Logrank} = (O_A - E_A)^2 \left(\frac{1}{E_A} + \frac{1}{E_B} \right) \tag{4.4}$$

since $(O_A - E_A)^2 = (O_B - E_B)^2$. This format provides a direct comparison with equation (4.11) below and is one which we shall use later.

4.3 THE HAZARD RATIO

From the calculations summarised in Table 4.3 we can obtain the ratio $O_A/E_A = 11/8.435382 = 1.304031$, which is an estimate of the hazard rate in group A.

The value being greater than unity suggests that there are more deaths in the treatment A group than would be expected under the null hypothesis of equal treatment efficacy. In contrast, patients receiving treatment B experience fewer deaths than expected. The hazard rate for them is $O_B/E_B = 5/7.564618 = 0.660972$. We can combine these rates into a single statistic which gives a useful summary of the results of a particular study. In particular, as shown in equation (1.5), we can calculate the hazard ratio (HR), defined as the ratio of these two hazard rates; i.e.

$$HR = \frac{O_A/E_A}{O_B/E_B}. \tag{4.5}$$

Example

For the 30 patients with cervical cancer

$$\begin{aligned} HR &= 1.304031/0.660972 \\ &= 1.972899 \\ &= 1.97. \end{aligned}$$

The final figure for the HR is rounded to two decimal places once the calculations are complete, to give sensible precision.

The HR = 1.97 suggests a hazard with treatment A and which is approximately double that of treatment B. Alternatively the HR could have been defined as the ratio $(O_B/E_B)/(O_A/E_A) = 0.660972/1.304031 = 0.5068$. In that case the result would be described as B having approximately half the hazard rate of treatment A. The choice of which to calculate is determined by the context in which the HR is to be used.

As already indicated, the HR of greater than unity emphasises the fact that the patients receiving A are dying at a faster rate than those who receive B. However, the logrank test suggested that this excess was not statistically significant, since the p-value = 0.2, implying that these data are not inconsistent with the null hypothesis value of HR = 1.

Example from the literature

McDiarmid *et al.* (1985) recorded the time to complete healing of bedsores in 40 hospitalised patients randomised, in a double blind trial, to ultrasound (US) or mock-ultrasound (mock-US) therapy. They give HR = 1.12, which expresses the ratio of the healing rates in the two groups, with $\chi^2_{Logrank} = 0.1$, df = 1, p-value = 0.8, in favour of US. However, the number of sores healed was only 18 since many patients were either discharged or died before complete healing could be observed, and so this trial does not provide reliable evidence that US is better than mock-US.

It is useful to summarise the results, following the calculation of the HR and the logrank test, in a tabular form similar to that of Table 4.5, which uses the data from the worked example for the 30 patients with cervical cancer.

Example from the literature

Nash *et al.* (1990) compared the value of high- as opposed to low-frequency

Table 4.5 Presentation of results following the logrank test of the worked example of the survival time of 30 patients with cervical cancer

Treatment	Number of patients (n)	Number of deaths		O/E	HR	$\chi^2_{Logrank}$	P
		Observed (O)	Expected (E)				
A	16	11	8.44	1.30			
					1.97	1.65	0.20
B	14	5	7.56	0.66			
Total	30	16	16.00				

transcutaneous electrical nerve stimulation (TENS) for the relief of pain in a randomised trial. They measured the time taken, from the date of randomisation for the patients to achieve a 50% reduction in pain levels as compared to those levels recorded at admission to the trial. Pain was measured using a visual analogue scale (VAS). The cumulative pain relief rates are summarised in Figure 4.5 and Table 4.6.

Of the 200 patients recruited—100 randomised to low-frequency and 100 to high-frequency TENS—only 55 achieved the reduction in pain defined as the critical event of interest. The HR = 1.41 suggests a considerable advantage of the high-frequency

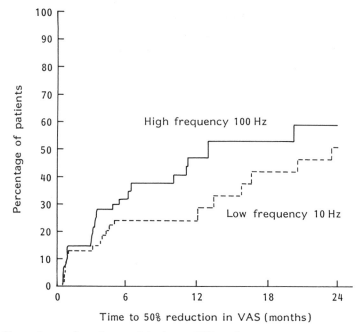

Figure 4.5 Percentage of patients achieving a 50% reduction in VAS for high- and low-frequency simulation (From Nash *et al.*, 1990. Reproduced by permission of VSP International Science Publishers.)

Table 4.6 Results of the trial comparing low and high frequency TENS (From Nash *et al.*, 1990. Reproduced by permission of VSP International Science Publishers.)

Frequency	Number of patients (n)	Number achieving relief		O/E	HR	$\chi^2_{Logrank}$	p
		Observed (O)	Expected (E)				
Low	100	24	28.7	0.84			
					1.41	1.64	0.20
High	100	31	26.3	1.18			
Total	200	55	55.0				

therapy. However, this does not reach conventional statistical significance ($\chi^2_{Logrank} = 1.64$, df = 1, p-value = 0.20). Clearly, the number of events observed is relatively small, and because of this, although the estimate of the treatment effect suggests high-frequency therapy may be of considerable benefit to patients, this trial has not been able to provide reliable evidence to support this.

Example from the literature

A useful format for the summary of the calculations of the logrank test and HR, together with the corresponding survival curves, is presented by Mufti *et al.* (1985) and is shown in Figure 4.6. Although they do not explicitly show the HR, this can be calculated as HR = 3.69/0.71 = 5.20. This shows a very adverse prognosis for patients with myelodysplastic syndromes with bone marrow blasts ≥5%. This is statistically significant with a p-value = 0.00001. They also quote the median survival times for the two patient groups as 9 and 39 months for those with <5% and ≥5% bone marrow blasts, respectively.

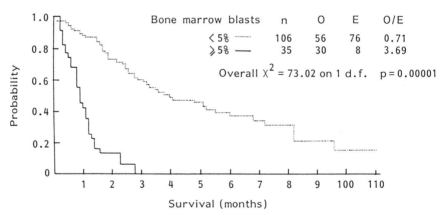

Figure 4.6 Survival in patients with myelodysplastic syndromes according to bone marrow blasts at presentation (From Mufti *et al.*, 1985. Reproduced by permission of *Br. J. Haematol.* 59: 425–33.)

4.4 CONFIDENCE INTERVALS FOR THE HAZARD RATIO

Whenever an estimate of a difference between groups is given, it is useful to calculate a confidence interval (CI) for the estimate. Thus, for the HR obtained from any trial, we would like to know a range of values which are not inconsistent with the observation.

In calculating CIs, it is convenient if the statistic under consideration can be assumed to follow an approximately Normal distribution. However, the estimate of the HR is not normally distributed. In particular it has a possible range of values from 0 to ∞, with the null hypothesis value of unity not located at the centre of this interval. To make the scale symmetric and to enable us to calculate CIs, we transform the estimate to make it approximately normally distributed. We do this by using log HR, rather than HR itself, as the basis for our calculation.

It is possible to show that a general $100(1 - \alpha)\%$ CI for the logarithm of the HR is given by

$$\log HR - [z_{1 - \alpha/2} \times SE(\log HR)] \quad \text{to} \quad \log HR + [z_{1 - \alpha/2} \times SE(\log HR)] \quad (4.6)$$

where $z_{1 - \alpha/2}$ is the upper $(1 - \alpha/2)$ point of the standard Normal distribution (see Figure 1.6). The $100(1 - \alpha)\%$ CI for the HR itself is then

$$\exp[\log HR - z_{1 - \alpha/2} SE(\log HR)] \quad \text{to} \quad \exp[\log HR + z_{1 - \alpha/2} SE(\log HR)]. \quad (4.7)$$

In both these expressions

$$SE(\log HR) = \sqrt{\left(\frac{1}{E_A} + \frac{1}{E_B}\right)}. \quad (4.8)$$

Example

For the data of Table 4.3, $E_A = 8.435382$, $E_B = 7.564618$ and therefore

$$SE(\log HR) = \sqrt{[(1/8.435382) + (1/7.564618)]}$$
$$= \sqrt{0.250743}$$
$$= 0.500742.$$

A 95% CI sets $z_{0.975} = 1.96$ and gives, from equation (4.6), a range from $0.6780 - 1.96 \times 0.500742$ to $0.6870 + 1.96 \times 0.500742$ or -0.3035 to 1.6595 as the interval. Finally, to obtain the CI for the HR we exponentiate these lower and upper limits, as in equation (4.7), to obtain 0.74 to 5.26.

This wide interval emphasises the inconclusive nature of the study in that the data are consistent both with a five-fold increase in hazard on treatment A, and also a reduction in the hazard with A of one quarter (1–0.74), as compared to those patients receiving treatment B. Although this is only an illustrative example, the 95% CI emphasizes that reliable conclusions cannot be drawn from these data.

Example from the literature

The full results of the trial in women with cervical cancer have been published by the MRC Working Party on Advanced Carcinoma of the Cervix (1993). They give

Table 4.7 Results from the logrank test for treatment differences on survival in patients with cervical cancer (From MRC Working Party on Advanced Carcinoma of the Cervix, 1993. Reproduced by permission of *Radiotherapy Oncology* 26: 93–103.)

Treatment*	Number of patients (n)	Number of events		O/E	HR	$\chi^2_{Logrank}$	p
		Observed (O)	Expected (E)				
RTX + Ro-8799	91	45	36.20	1.24			
					1.58	4.05	0.044
RTX alone	92	32	40.80	0.78			
	183	77	77.00				

*Note the treatments are presented in reverse order to our illustration in Table 4.5.

for 183 patients randomised either to receive radiotherapy alone or radiotherapy plus a sensitizer (Ro-8799), the logrank test, HR and associated CI using survival as the endpoint. Their results are summarised in Table 4.7. The 95% CI for the HR is 1.01 to 2.48 which (just) excludes the null hypothesis value of 1.

Table 4.7 shows that only 77 (42%) of patients had died at the time of this analysis, which suggests that a more statistically powerful comparison of these treatments could have been obtained if analysis had been delayed. In fact the MRC Working Party on Advanced Carcinoma of the Cervix (1993) indicated this as an interim analysis of these data. The reasons for this interim, rather than final, analysis are discussed in detail by Parmar and Machin (1993).

Example from the literature

Nash *et al.* (1990), in the example described earlier in Table 4.6 and Figure 4.5, give an HR = 1.41 and a 95% CI for the HR as 0.8 to 2.6. This interval includes HR = 1, the value we would expect if there was no difference between the two frequencies in their effect on pain relief. However, the interval is also consistent with, for example, HR = 2 or a large benefit of the high-frequency therapy.

4.5   THE MANTEL–HAENSZEL TEST

The estimate of the SE(log HR) given in equation (4.8) is not always reliable in situations when the total number of events in the study is small. A preferred estimate of the SE, albeit involving more extensive computation, requires the calculation of the variance, called the hypergeometric variance, at each death time. Summing these variances across all times leads to the Mantel–Haenszel version of the logrank test.

Referring back to Table 4.4 the hypergeometric variance at time t is given by

$$V_t = \frac{m_t n_t r_t s_t}{N_t^2 (N_t - 1)}. \tag{4.9}$$

If all deaths occur at different times, i.e. there are no tied observations, then $r_t = 1$, $s_t = N_t - 1$ and equation (4.9) simplifies to

$$V_t = m_t n_t / N_t^2.$$

The calculation of V_t at each time point, t, is shown in Table 4.3, for 30 of the patients recruited to the cervical cancer trial. The general calculation of V_t from equation (4.9) is repeated in the lower panel of Table 4.4.

As for both E_{At} and E_{Bt}, we finally sum the individual V_t calculated at each distinct event time to obtain

$$V = \Sigma \ V_t. \tag{4.10}$$

The Mantel–Haenszel test statistic is then defined as

$$\chi^2_{MH} = \frac{(O_A - E_A)^2}{V}. \tag{4.11}$$

As for the logrank test of equation (4.3), the Mantel–Haenszel test statistic has an approximate χ^2 distribution with one degree of freedom. It should be noted that χ^2_{MH} of equation (4.11) only differs from $\chi^2_{Logrank}$ of equation (4.4) by the expression for V.

It should also be noted that the numerator of equation (4.11) can be replaced by the corresponding expression for treatment B, since for the two-group comparison considered here, as $(O_B - E_B) = -(O_A - E_A)$. The difference in sign is removed once the square is taken. In fact, it can be shown that the individual components of the numerator of equation (4.11) are $(O_{At} - E_{At})^2 = (n_t O_{At} - m_t O_{Bt})^2$. This format illustrates the symmetry of equation (4.11) with respect to treatments A and B more clearly.

Example

Using the calculations from Table 4.3 we have $O_A = 11$, $E_A = 8.435382$, $V = 3.910995$ and therefore from equation (4.11) we have

$$\chi^2_{MH} = (2.564618)^2 / 3.910995$$
$$= 1.681737.$$

This is very similar to $\chi^2_{Logrank} = 1.649201$ obtained earlier using equation (4.3) and, in this example, the extra calculation required for the Mantel–Haenszel statistic is hardly justified. However, in certain circumstances, especially if there are many ties in the data, the difference between the two can be much larger.

The use of the Mantel–Haenszel statistic to test for the difference between two groups also gives an alternative estimate of the HR. This estimate is

$$HR_{MH} = \exp\left(\frac{O_A - E_A}{V}\right). \tag{4.12}$$

This contrasts with that given by equation (4.5).

Example

Using the HR estimator of equation (4.12) gives, for the data of Table 4.3. $O_A - E_A = 2.564618$, $V = 3.910995$ and

$$
\begin{aligned}
HR_{MH} &= \exp(2.564618/3.910995) \\
&= \exp(0.655746) \\
&= 1.9266 \\
&= 1.93.
\end{aligned}
$$

This is very close to the HR = 1.97 that we obtained using equation (4.5). Thus the two seemingly quite different estimates of the HR give almost identical results. As already indicated, if there are ties in the data the estimates will diverge but, except in rather unusual circumstances, they will usually be close to each other. In fact if there are no ties in the data, as is the case in our example, the two methods lead to the same value except for rounding errors introduced by the different methods of calculation.

The corresponding SE of the Mantel–Haenszel log HR_{MH} is

$$
SE(\log HR_{MH}) = 1/V^{1/2}. \tag{4.13}
$$

Example

For the example in Table 4.3 equation (4.13) gives

$$
SE(\log HR_{MH}) = 1/\sqrt{(3.910995)} = 0.505657.
$$

This is very close to the previous value given by equation (4.8), which was 0.500742.

The SE of log HR_{MH} given in equation (4.13) can be used together with equation (4.12) in expression (4.7) to give CIs derived from the Mantel–Haenszel estimate of the HR as

$$
\exp[\log HR_{MH} - (z_{1-\alpha/2}/V^{1/2})] \text{ to } \exp[\log HR_{MH} + (z_{1-\alpha/2}/V^{1/2})]. \tag{4.14}
$$

As the values obtained of log HR_{MH} and $SE(\log HR_{MH})$, respectively, in our example are so close to those obtained earlier, the numerical calculation of the CI using equation (4.14) is omitted.

4.6   THE STRATIFIED LOGRANK TEST

As we have indicated earlier, in any clinical study the outcome for patients may be as much, if not more, influenced by characteristics of the patients themselves as by the treatments they receive. In contraceptive development trials, for example, cultural considerations may influence the continuation of use of new contraceptives as much as the 'efficacy' of the method itself. In cancer, it is well known that patients with a more advanced stage of the disease have a shorter expectation of life than patients with less advanced disease. Thus, patients with Stage III cervical cancer will (on average) do worse than those with Stage IIb. When making comparisons between two groups receiving, for example, different treatments, we need to ensure as much as possible that the differences observed between groups is due to the treatments and not due to the fact that the groups have inherently differing prognoses. We thus may wish to adjust for these prognostic variables when making comparisons between groups. In a trial of two treatments (A and B) in women with cervical cancer we can do this by first making a comparison of treatment A against treatment B within each cervical cancer stage separately. This ensures that 'like' is compared with 'like'. These individual comparisons are then combined to achieve an overall comparison of treatments. This is done by means of the stratified logrank test.

To illustrate the method, stage of disease for each patient with cervical cancer is added, in Table 4.8, to the data previously outlined in Table 4.2. For example, the patient who died after 90 days had Stage III disease. The calculation of the stratified logrank test proceeds exactly as that described earlier in Table 4.3, but first confining the comparison to within one of the strata. The first strata analysis is summarised in the Stage IIb section of Table 4.9. A similar analysis is then made within the second strata, here Stage III. Thus for the stratum of Stage IIb patients, $O_A = 3$, $E_A = 2.105129$, $O_B = 1$ and $E_B = 1.894871$, while for the stratum of Stage III disease the corresponding values are $O_A = 8$, $E_A = 7.813810$, $O_B = 4$ and $E_B = 4.186190$. The next step is to combine the stratum-specific observed and expected values across the two strata, to obtain

$$\sum_s O_A = 3 + 8 = 11, \qquad \sum_s E_A = 2.105129 + 7.813810 = 9.918939$$

$$\sum_z O_B = 1 + 4 = 5, \qquad \sum_s E_B = 1.894871 + 4.186190 = 6.081061$$

Table 4.8 Ranked survival times by disease stage and treatment in 30 patients with cervical cancer

	Control A				New therapy B		
Patient number	Stage	Survival time	Survival status	Patient number	Stage	Survival time	Survival status
11	III	90	DEAD	28	III	272	DEAD
15	III	142	DEAD	25	III	362	DEAD
23	III	150	DEAD	16	III	373	DEAD
29	III	269	DEAD	27	III	383+	ALIVE
6	IIb	291	DEAD	7	III	519+	ALIVE
30	IIb	468+	ALIVE	18	III	563+	ALIVE
5	III	680	DEAD	22	III	650+	ALIVE
24	III	837	DEAD	3	III	827	DEAD
26	IIb	890+	ALIVE	13	IIb	919+	ALIVE
2	III	1037	DEAD	21	IIb	978+	ALIVE
14	IIb	1090+	ALIVE	8	IIb	1100+	ALIVE
19	III	1113+	ALIVE	10	IIb	1307	DEAD
20	IIb	1153	DEAD	12	IIb	1360+	ALIVE
17	III	1297	DEAD	1	IIb	1476+	ALIVE
4	IIb	1429	DEAD				
9	IIb	1577+	ALIVE				

Table 4.9 Stratified logrank test for comparison of treatments A with B in patients with cervical cancer adjusted for stage of the disease

Patient number	Rank	Survival (days) A	B		Dead	Alive	Total	E_{At}	E_{Bt}	V_t
Stage IIb										
6	1	291		A	1	6	7			
				B	0	6	6			
					1	12	13	0.538462	0.461538	0.248520
30	2	468+								
26	3	890+								
13	4		919+							
21	5		978+							
14	6	1090+								
8	7		1100+							
20	8	1153		A	1	2	3			
				B	0	3	3			
					1	5	6	0.500000	0.500000	0.250000
10	9		1307	A	0	2	2			
				B	1	2	3			
					1	4	5	0.400000	0.600000	0.240000
12	10		1360+							
4	11	1429		A	1	1	2			
				B	0	1	1			
					1	2	3	0.666667	0.333333	0.222222
1	12		1476+							
9	13	1577+								

			Total	$O_A = 3$ $O_B = 1$ $E_A = 2.105129$ $E_B = 1.894871$ $V = 0.960742$

Patient number	Rank	Survival (days) A	B		Dead	Alive	Total	E_{At}	E_{Bt}	V_t
Stage III										
11	1	90		A	1	8	9			
				B	0	8	8			
					1	16	17	0.529412	0.470588	0.249135
15	2	142		A	1	7	8			
				B	0	8	8			
					1	15	16	0.500000	0.500000	0.250000
23	3	150		A	1	6	7			
				B	0	8	8			
					1	14	15	0.466667	0.533333	0.248889
29	4	269		A	1	5	6			
				B	0	8	8			
					1	13	14	0.428571	0.571429	0.244899

Table 4.9 (*continued*)

Patient number	Rank	Survival (days) A	B		Dead	Alive	Total	E_{At}	E_{Bt}	V_t
28	5		272	A	0	5	5			
				B	1	7	8			
					1	12	13	0.384615	0.615385	0.236686
25	6		362	A	0	5	5			
				B	1	6	7			
					1	11	12	0.416667	0.583333	0.243056
16	7		373	A	0	5	5			
				B	1	5	6			
					1	10	11	0.454545	0.545455	0.247934
27	8		383+							
7	9		519+							
18	10		563+							
22	11		650+							
5	12	680		A	1	4	5			
				B	0	1	1			
					1	5	6	0.833333	0.166667	0.138888
3	13		827	A	0	4	4			
				B	1	0	1			
					1	4	5	0.800000	0.200000	0.160000
24	14	837		A	1	3	4			
				B	0	0	0			
					1	3	4	1.000000	0.000000	0.000000
2	15	1037		A	1	2	3			
				B	0	0	0			
					1	2	3	1.000000	0.000000	0.000000
19	16	1113+								
17	17	1297		A	1	0	1			
				B	0	0	0			
					1	0	1	1.000000	0.000000	0.000000

Total $O_A = 8$ $O_B = 4$ $E_A = 7.813810$ $E_B = 4.186190$ $V = 2.019478$

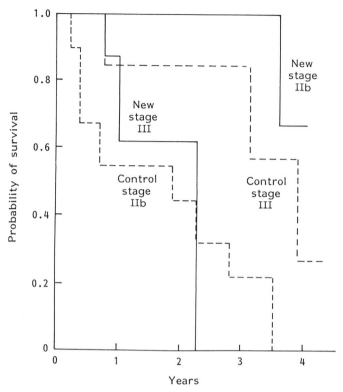

Figure 4.7   Survival for patients with cervical cancer by the four stage by treatment groups

Here s beneath the Σ denotes the sum over the strata. The stratified HR_s is then given by

$$HR_S = \left(\sum_s O_A \middle/ \sum_s E_A\right) \middle/ \left(\sum_s O_B \middle/ \sum_s E_B\right)$$

$$= \frac{(11/9.918939)}{(5/6.081061)} = \frac{1.1090}{0.8222} = 1.3488. \tag{4.15}$$

In this example, HR_s, the stratified or adjusted HR, is less than $HR = 1.97$ calculated earlier in Table 4.5. This suggests that there is an imbalance of patients with Stages IIb and III in the respective treatment groups. This has clearly affected the comparison between the two treatment groups in a serious way. The corresponding Kaplan–Meier survival curves for the four stage by treatment groups are shown in Figure 4.7.

By analogy with equation (4.3) the stratified logrank statistic for comparing treatments is

$$\chi^2_{\text{Stratified}} = \frac{\left(\sum_s O_A - \sum_s E_A\right)^2}{\sum_s E_A} + \frac{\left(\sum_s O_B - \sum_s E_B\right)^2}{\sum_s E_B}. \tag{4.16}$$

We have included the s denoting the sum over the strata here to aid clarity but it is often omitted. This also has a χ^2 distribution with $df = 1$ since we are comparing two treatments A and B.

Example

For the patients with Stage IIb and III cervical cancer we have, using equation (4.16), for the stratified logrank test

$$\chi^2_{Stratified} = \frac{(11 - 9.918939)^2}{9.918939} + \frac{(5 - 6.081061)^2}{6.081061}$$

$$= 0.310010.$$

This contrasts with $\chi^2_{Logrank} = 1.649201$ derived from the unadjusted logrank test calculated earlier.

In randomised trials with large numbers of patients it would be unusual to see such a difference in value between the adjusted and unadjusted analyses. However, in non-randomised or smaller randomised trials, large differences between adjusted and unadjusted analyses can be expected. In these instances adjusted analyses are usually performed and reported.

4.7 MEDIAN SURVIVAL

If M_1 and M_2 are the respective median survival times of two groups calculated as indicated in chapter 2.6, then an estimate of the HR can be obtained from

$$HR_{Median} = M_2/M_1. \tag{4.17}$$

In this case, it is the inverse of the ratio of the two medians that estimates the HR for group 1 as compared to group 2.

A CI for this HR is given by

$$\exp\{\log (M_2/M_1) - \{z_{1-\alpha/2} \times SE[\log(M_2/M_1)]\}\}$$

to

$$\exp\{\log (M_2/M_1) + \{z_{1-\alpha/2} \times SE[\log(M_2/M_1)]\}\}. \tag{4.18}$$

Here the SE is given by

$$SE(\log M_2/M_1) = \sqrt{[(1/O_1) + (1/O_2)]} \tag{4.19}$$

where O_1 and O_2 are the observed numbers of deaths in the two groups.

This method of estimating the HR and the associated CI assumes an exponential distribution (chapter 3) for the survival times and is therefore seldom used in practice. France et al. (1991) report on the use of a CI for the difference between two medians rather than their ratio.

Example

Reading the median survival times of patients with cervical cancer from Figure 4.2 for the two treatment groups with corresponding deaths $O_A = 11$ and $O_B = 5$ gives $M_A = 1037$ and $M_B = 1307$ days.

Hence from equation (4.17) the $HR_{Median} = M_B/M_A = 1307/1037 = 1.2604$. This gives $\log HR_{Median} = \log (1.2604) = 0.2314$ and the SE $(\log HR_{Median}) = \sqrt{[(1/11) + (1/5)]} = 0.5394$. The 95% CI for this estimated HR is therefore $\exp[0.2314 - (1.96 \times 0.5394)]$ to $\exp[0.2314 + (1.96 \times 0.5394)]$, i.e. $\exp(-0.825824) = 0.4379$ to $\exp(1.288624) = 3.6278$ or 0.4 to 3.6. The width of the CI reflects the considerable uncertainty about the value of the HR.

4.8 NON-PROPORTIONAL HAZARDS

GRAPHICAL ASSESSMENT OF PROPORTIONAL HAZARDS

We have described in section 4.2 the logrank test and in section 4.5 the Mantel–Haenszel test for comparing two survival curves. These two tests are statistically the most powerful in assessing differences between two survival curves when the ratio of the hazard rates (hazards) for the two groups are approximately constant as time progresses. In this case, the hazards are termed proportional. Proportional hazards are discussed in more detail below and in chapter 7. In circumstances when the hazards are not proportional, the tests can still be used, but they may not be the most powerful tests available. Thus, in instances in which non-proportional hazards are *anticipated*, it may be better to use alternative methods of analysis.

We described in chapter 3 a method of assessing whether the hazard within a particular group remains constant with time. An illustration, using data of patients with colorectal cancer, is given in Figure 3.4. This method can be extended to assessing constancy of the ratio of the relative hazards in two patient groups by calculating such a plot for the two groups separately. This involves plotting $\log\{-\log [S(t)]\}$ against log t for each group.

Example

Figure 4.8 shows the $\log\{-\log [S(t)]\}$ against log t plots for two groups of patients with a brain cancer. One group of patients had a history of fits prior to diagnosis and the other group did not. From Figure 4.8 we can see that the hazard is approximately constant within each group, as each plot is approximately linear. The two lines are approximately parallel, which indicates a constant ratio of relative hazards between the two groups as time progresses. This in turn suggests that an overall summary by use of the HR is likely to be appropriate.

In contrast Figure 4.9 shows the same type of plot for the patients contributing to Figure 4.8 but now divided into three groups on the basis of their age.

From this plot we see that although the relative hazards for the 45–59 and 60+ years groups are approximately constant, they are not proportional, as the two lines

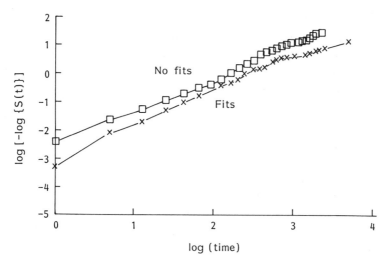

Figure 4.8 Graph of log {−log[S(t)]} against log t in two groups of patients with brain tumours (From Medical Research Council Working Party on Misonidazole in Gliomas, 1983. Reproduced by permission of The British Institute of Radiology.)

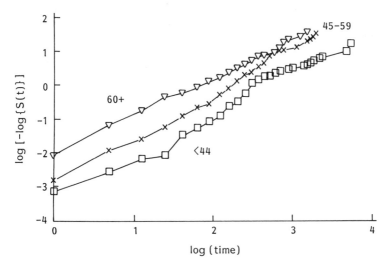

Figure 4.9 Graph of log {−log[S(t)]} against log t in three age groups of patients with brain tumours (From Medical Research Council Working Party on Misonidazole in Gliomas, 1983. Reproduced by permission of The British Institute of Radiology.)

converge as time increases. There is also a suggestion that the hazard for the younger patients does not appear to be constant, since there is some suggestion of a flattening of the plot for values of log t greater than 2.5. Thus, comparing the three groups, it would appear that the assumption of proportional hazards may not be appropriate, particularly for the comparison of the 45–59 and 60+ age groups.

Example from the literature

Nolan *et al.* (1991) give the time to remission from incontinence in a randomised trial of two laxatives. They compare a multimodal therapy (MM) and behaviour modification only (BM), in 169 children: 86 receiving BM and 83 MM. The Kaplan–Meier estimates of the corresponding remission from incontinence times of the two groups are shown in Figure 4.10. In this example, the lower survival curve indicates an advantage to that therapy, as patients receiving that therapy have a faster remission of their incontinence.

The two Kaplan–Meier curves cross at approximately 70 weeks, with an apparent advantage to the MM group prior to this time and thereafter a disadvantage. In this situation the complementary log plots would also cross, suggesting that the relative hazards do not remain proportional. However, it should be stressed here that the curves become less reliable with time so that the crossing at 70 weeks could merely be a consequence of small numbers of events observed in that region.

WEIGHTED MANTEL–HAENSZEL TESTS

A number of tests have been proposed which compare two survival curves for the non-proportional hazards situation. These tests can be generated from one basic formula and are known as weighted Mantel–Haenszel tests. For a two-group comparison of A and B, these are defined as

$$\chi^2_{MHw} = \frac{\sum w_t (O_{At} - E_{At})^2}{\sum w_t^2 V_{At}}. \tag{4.20}$$

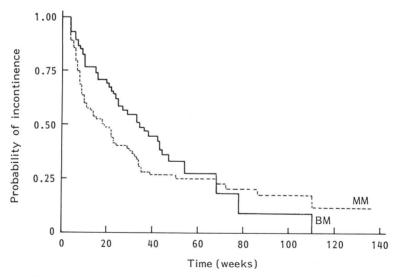

Figure 4.10 Kaplan–Meier curves for time to remission from incontinence by treatment group (From Nolan *et al.*, 1991, Randomised trials of laxatives in treatment of childhood encopresis, Lancet 338, 523–527, © by The Lancet Ltd, 1991)

Here, E_{At} and V_{At} are calculated as described by equations (4.1) and (4.9), respectively. The weights are the w_t and can vary as time, t, changes. These tests all give a statistic which is distributed as χ^2 with df = 1 for the two group comparisons discussed here.

If we set $w_t = 1$, for all values of t, then this assigns equal weight to each death at whatever time, t, it occurs. In this situation, equation (4.20) becomes that of the (unweighted) Mantel–Haenszel test of equation (4.11). This is the most powerful test when the hazards are (approximately) proportional.

If we set $w_t \neq 1$ we are implicitly stating that differences between certain parts of the survival curves being compared are of greater interest than others. For example, if it is anticipated that a new treatment may help avoid the particular risk of early deaths when compared with the standard treatment but thereafter holds no particular advantage, then extra weight may be assigned to any early deaths. One way in which this can be achieved is by setting $w_t = R_t$, where R_t is the total number of patients at risk at time, t, as we have described in chapter 2.8 and equation (2.11). In most examples, this number declines over time, t, as the total number of deaths and censored observations increases with time. This test, therefore, places greater emphasis or weight on 'earlier' parts of the curves. This version of the test is known as the Gehan, generalised Wilcoxon or Breslow test, and is

$$\chi^2_G = \frac{\sum R_t(O_{At} - E_{At})^2}{\sum R_t^2 V_t}. \tag{4.21}$$

To calculate χ^2_G it is necessary to calculate the components of both the numerator and denominator at each death time, as was done in Table 4.3, to obtain O_{At}, E_{At} and V_t.

Example from the literature

Nolan *et al.* (1991) quote both the Mantel–Haenszel version of logrank test with p-value = 0.12, corresponding to $\chi^2_{MH} = 0.82$, df = 1, and the Gehan test, with p-value = 0.012, corresponding to $\chi^2_G = 6.30$, df = 1. They also comment that 'The proportionality assumption was not satisfied for the full follow-up period'.

The difference in the p-values given by the two tests leads to quite different interpretations of the data and demonstrates how important it is to plot the survival curves for the two groups so that an appropriate interpretation of the significance tests can be made.

Care must be taken in applying the Gehan test as it can be very misleading when there are many censored observations or when the censoring is unequal in the two groups. These situations can arise in the early life of a prospective study, for example in a clinical trial which is still in the recruitment phase. In this case there may be many patients recently entered and therefore insufficient observation time for the critical events to occur. Unequal censoring can occur if, for whatever reason, information is systematically received on events occurring earlier in one group than in the other. For example, in a randomised trial to compare patients using a regular and predetermined appointments system against a system in which patients present only when they notice symptoms of recurrence, one could argue that those patients with fixed appointments will be examined more rigorously and early signs of recurrence thus detected and reported. In contrast, patients assigned to the other group will only report recurrence once the symptoms are clearly obvious to the patient.

A similar but less extreme means of weighting the earlier part of the survival curve, than through the Gehan test, is given by using the Tarone–Ware version of equation (4.20). This is

$$\chi^2_{TW} = \frac{\sum R_t^{1/2}(O_{At} - E_{At})^2}{\sum R_t V_t} \qquad (4.22)$$

where the w_t of equation (4.19) are set equal to $R_t^{1/2}$. This still gives more weight to the early deaths observed in the study but in a less extreme way than that of equation (4.21).

A further set of weights has been suggested by both Peto and Prentice. Their test is

$$\chi^2_{PP} = \frac{\sum w_{PPt}(O_{At} - E_{At})^2}{\sum w_{PPt} V_t} \qquad (4.23)$$

where

$$w_{PPt} = \prod_{j=1}^{t} \frac{(R_j - d_j + 1)}{(R_j + 1)}.$$

Here d_j is the number of events at time j. The weighting for this χ^2_{PP} test is similar to the corresponding estimate of the Kaplan–Meier survival curve at each event given by equation (2.5) but with n_j replaced by $R_j + 1$. The aim of these weights is similar to both the Gehan and Tarone–Ware weights, in that the earlier parts of the curves are given greater weighting than the later sections.

Example

Using the data from 30 patients with cervical cancer analysed in Table 4.3 the calculation of the various χ^2 statistics for the Mantel–Haenszel, Gehan, Tarone–Ware and Peto–Prentice tests are summarised in Table 4.10. For brevity of presentation, the censored survival times are omitted and the death times for both treatments A and B are ranked together in the first column of the table, but with death times for treatment A indicated in bold.

For all the tests we only have to calculate the contribution to the test statistic at each death time. In Table 4.10 the actual weight, w_t, with each method is presented, together with the relative weight W_t, which is the weight at time t divided by the sum of all the weights, for each death, i.e. $W_t = w_t / \sum w_t$. The latter is given because it allows more direct comparisons between the different statistical test weights, given to each death. Thus, for example, we see that the Mantel–Haenszel method gives the first death at time 90 days (at the earliest part

Table 4.10 Weights (w_t) and relative weights (W_t) for four weighted Mantel–Haenszel tests applied to survival data from 30 patients with cervical cancer

Death time (t)	$O_{At} - E_{At}$	V_t	Mantel–Haenszel w_t	Mantel–Haenszel W_t	Gehan R_t	Gehan W_t	Tarone–Ware $R_t^{1/2}$	Tarone–Ware W_t	Peto-Prentice w_{PPt}	Peto-Prentice W_t
90[a]	0.46667	0.24889	1	0.0625	30	0.1027	5.47723	0.0836	0.96774	0.0886
142	0.48276	0.25000	1	0.0625	29	0.0993	5.38517	0.0822	0.93548	0.0857
150	0.50000	0.25000	1	0.0625	28	0.0959	5.29150	0.0808	0.90323	0.0827
269	0.51852	0.24966	1	0.0625	27	0.0925	5.19615	0.0793	0.87097	0.0798
272	−0.46154	0.24852	1	0.0625	26	0.0890	5.09902	0.0778	0.83871	0.0768
291	0.52000	0.24960	1	0.0625	25	0.0856	5.00000	0.0763	0.80645	0.0739
362	−0.45833	0.24826	1	0.0625	24	0.0822	4.89898	0.0748	0.77419	0.0709
373	−0.47826	0.24953	1	0.0625	23	0.0788	4.79583	0.0732	0.74194	0.0679
680	0.41177	0.24222	1	0.0625	17	0.0582	4.12311	0.0629	0.70072	0.0642
827	−0.56250	0.24609	1	0.0625	16	0.0548	4.00000	0.0611	0.65950	0.0604
837	0.40000	0.24000	1	0.0625	15	0.0514	3.87298	0.0591	0.61828	0.0566
1037	0.36364	0.23141	1	0.0625	11	0.0377	3.31663	0.0516	0.56676	0.0519
1153	0.42857	0.24490	1	0.0625	7	0.0240	2.64575	0.0404	0.49591	0.0454
1297	0.50000	0.25000	1	0.0625	6	0.0206	2.44949	0.0374	0.42507	0.0389
1307	−0.40000	0.24000	1	0.0625	5	0.0171	2.23607	0.0341	0.35422	0.0324
1429	0.33333	0.22222	1	0.0625	3	0.0103	1.73205	0.0264	0.26567	0.0243
Total	2.564586	3.910995	16	1	292	1	65.62	1	10.92	1

[a] The death time in bold correspond to deaths on treatment A, the remainder treatment B.

of the curve) a weight of 6.25%, while the Gehan, Tarone–Ware and Peto–Prentice tests give weights of 10.27%, 8.36%, and 8.86%, respectively, to this first death. In contrast, if we consider the last death at 1429 days the relative weights for the four tests are 6.25%, 1.03%, 2.64% and 2.43%, respectively. Of all the tests, the Mantel–Haenszel statistic gives the most weight to the tail end of the curves. This is a weight equal to that for all other deaths, whenever they occur. In contrast, the Gehan test gives the least weight amongst these four tests to the longest surviving patients.

The corresponding χ^2 statistics for the four tests are summarised in Table 4.11, together, for completeness, with that for the logrank test. In this example, all five tests give rather similar results. It is important to emphasise that, whatever test is used, it should be specified at the design stage of the study, i.e. before the data are collected and analysed. Any test specified either after the data are collected or as a consequence of inspection of the resulting Kaplan–Meier survival curves must be regarded as secondary or exploratory. Such 'data-snooping' tests should be interpreted with great care for the presence of spurious statistical significance. In practice, it will often be very difficult to anticipate the shape of the survival curves with any degree of certainty. In such situations, and in general therefore, the Mantel–Haenszel version of the logrank test is recommended for the primary analysis.

Table 4.11 χ^2 statistics and p-values from the application of the logrank, Mantel–Haenszel and weighted tests for the data of Table 4.3

Statistical test	χ^2	p-value
Logrank	1.649	0.2005
Mantel–Haenszel (MH)	1.682	0.1947
Gehan (G)	1.292	0.2380
Tarone–Ware (TW)	1.513	0.2186
Peto–Prentice (PP)	1.742	0.1869

4.9   COMPARING FOLLOW-UP IN TWO GROUPS

We described in section 2.12 a method of summarising the maturity of the follow-up data for a single patient group. This method can be extended to two or more groups by use of the Kaplan–Meier plots of the follow-up curves. These curves can be visually compared to assess any differences and the corresponding median, minimum and maximum follow-up in the groups obtained.

If we return to the situation of comparing two or more *survival* curves, we usually assume that the censoring mechanisms do not depend on the group. For example, in a randomised clinical trial, it is assumed that patients are just as likely to be lost to follow-up in one treatment group as in the other. In contrast, if one is comparing new patients with a historical series, one might expect, since the new patient set is less mature, a greater proportion of censored data in this group. These censored data are not necessarily lost to follow-up but are made up of subjects that are currently being followed at the time of analysis or census date.

Such imbalances in follow-up can lead to a spurious difference in survival between groups. In the context of a randomised trial any imbalance in follow-up, for whatever reason, is likely to be important. This is particularly the case at an interim analysis when only relatively few events, of the total anticipated by the design, have been observed. Such an imbalance in follow-up between the treatment groups could lead to the spurious conclusion that there is a difference in the survival patterns in the groups. Thus, any survival comparisons between groups, whether final or interim, should always be accompanied by a comparison of the follow-up in the groups being compared. A simple way of doing this is to form the Kaplan–Meier follow-up curves as described in section 2.12. Nevertheless, such follow-up curves have to be interpreted with care. For example, if in a randomised trial aimed at assessing the difference between two treatments one treatment is considerably more effective in preventing death than the other, we would anticipate a difference in the patterns in the follow-up curves. This occurs even if there is, in truth, no difference in follow-up, simply because the attrition in follow-up will be greater in one treatment arm than the other, as a consequence of the shorter survival times in one group. This problem will not be important if the difference between treatments is relatively small.

At an interim analysis a check for similar follow-up is particularly important, since we could anticipate seeing 'large' differences. A simple solution to this difficulty is to exclude those patients who have died and to form follow-up curves just for those patients who are left alive. Minimum, maximum and median follow-up times can then be read from these curves in the usual way. When there are a high proportion of deaths the Kaplan–Meier follow-up curves obtained in this way will obviously be relatively unstable, since these curves include only those patients still alive. However, if a high proportion of deaths have been observed, a comparison of the follow-up in the two groups is probably not so important.

Example

In a trial of the value of postoperative radiotherapy in patients with non-small cell lung cancer, the MRC Lung Cancer Working Party randomised 308 patients to receive either surgery followed by radiotherapy (SR) or surgery alone (S). The follow-up curves by allocated treatment group for the 44 patients remaining alive are shown in Figure 4.11. It can be seen that there is no obvious difference between the two groups.

The minimum is given by the time of the first event, the median by the 50th percentile and the maximum by the time of the last event. These are 1, 18 and 36 months, respectively, for the S group and 2, 21 and 36 months for the SR group of patients. These are clearly very similar for both treatment groups.

In cases where there does appear to be a difference in follow-up curves between groups, any differences in survival between of the two groups should be interpreted with care.

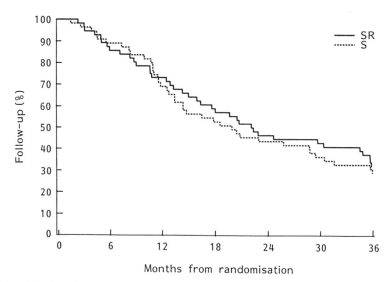

Figure 4.11 Kaplan–Meier estimates of 'follow-up' in two groups of patients (data provided by the Medical Research Council Lung Cancer Working Party)

4.10 TECHNICAL DETAILS

The standard χ^2 statistic of equation (1.14) is of the form $(O - E)^2/E$. It utilises a comparison of an observed statistic (O) minus its expected value (E) under the null hypothesis. This is divided by a variance term which, in this case, is also equal to E. For a 2×2 contingency table comparing two binomial proportions, such as the proportions of patients who respond to pirenzepine and trithiozine of Table 1.3, the test can be written as $\chi^2 = N(ad - bc)^2/mnrs$. This, in turn, can be expressed as $\chi^2 = [a - (rm/N)]^2/(mnrs/N^3)$.

The divisor in this latter expression is almost the (so called) hypergeometric variance $V = (mnrs)/[N^2(N-1)]$ of Table 4.4 except that $N-1$ is replaced by N. This similarity motivates the use of V in the Mantel–Haenszel test as we have indicated by equation (4.9).

This variance term is the same for both groups A and B. More formally we can write this as

$$V = Var(A) = Var(B) = \frac{mnrs}{N^2(N-1)}. \tag{4.24}$$

To generalise the Mantel–Haenszel test to more than two groups it is necessary to calculate the covariance of all the corresponding (pairs) of groups. The covariance of A and B, although not used explicitly in a two-group comparison, is

$$Cov(A, B) = -\frac{mnrs}{N^2(N-1)}. \tag{4.25}$$

5　More than Two Groups

Summary

This chapter describes how the logrank test can be extended to the comparison of
three or more groups. For situations where there is a natural ordering of the groups
a test for trend is described. The particular situation of a factorial design structure
for the groups is included. The Mantel–Haenszel alternative to the logrank test for
a three-group comparison is also described.

5.1　INTRODUCTION

We have described in chapter 4 how two groups may be compared using the
logrank test. There are also situations where we may wish to compare more than
two treatment groups in a clinical trial or compare outcomes for patients with
differing characteristics. For example, we may wish to compare the survival times
of patients with colon cancer by Dukes' stage A, B or C. This chapter describes how
the logrank test can be extended to three or more group comparisons. Of special
interest is the case where there is a factorial structure to the design or a natural
ordering of the groups under consideration.

5.2　THREE OR MORE GROUPS

Consider the data for the 30 women with cervical cancer that we have discussed
earlier (see Tables 4.1 and 4.2) whose age at diagnosis is presented by treatment
group in Table 5.1. For purposes of illustration we divide these women into three

Table 5.1   Age, age group and survival of 30 patients with cervical cancer by treatment group

	Control A				New Therapy B		
Patient number	Age (years)	Age group	Survival (days)	Patient number	Age (years)	Age group	Survival (days)
2	64	S	1037	1	63	S	1476+
4	69	S	1429	3	43	Y	827
5	38	Y	680	7	27	Y	519+
6	53	M	291	8	74	S	1100+
9	61	S	1577+	10	63	S	1307
11	59	M	90	12	39	Y	1360+
14	53	M	1090+	13	70	S	919+
15	56	M	142	16	68	S	373
17	65	S	1297	18	69	S	563+
19	48	Y	1113+	21	73	S	978+
20	45	Y	1153	22	58	M	650+
23	55	M	150	25	55	M	362
24	58	M	837	27	58	M	383+
26	49	Y	890+	28	45	Y	272
29	43	Y	269				
30	42	Y	468+				

groups according to age, and for convenience label them as young (less than 50), middle aged (50 to less than 60) and senior (60 or more) in an obvious notation of Y, M and S. The corresponding Kaplan–Meier plots are shown in Figure 5.1. In this small data set, the 11 older women (S) fare the best, the nine middle aged (M) the worst and the youngest 10 women (Y) intermediately.

The logrank comparison for these three groups (Y, M, S) proceeds in a similar way to the two-group comparison of Tables 4.3 and 4.4. Thus, the patients are first ordered by their survival times, as before, but now in three rows, one for each age group. At each death the data are summarised in a 3×2 contingency table, the first of which is shown in the upper panel of Table 5.2.

The full calculations are summarised in Table 5.3, from which it can be seen that, for example, $n_Y = 10$, $O_Y = 5$ and $E_Y = 4.610203$. The corresponding expression for the logrank statistic is an extension of equation (4.3) to three groups:

$$\chi^2_{\text{Logrank}} = \frac{(O_Y - E_Y)^2}{E_Y} + \frac{(O_M - E_M)^2}{E_M} + \frac{(O_S - E_S)^2}{E_S}. \qquad (5.1)$$

The general expression corresponding to equation (5.1), but for G groups, is given by

$$\chi^2_{\text{Logrank}} = \sum_{g=1}^{G} \frac{(O_g - E_g)^2}{E_g}. \qquad (5.2)$$

The calculated value of χ^2_{Logrank} has to be referred to Table T3, but with the corresponding degrees of freedom. In the case of G groups the degrees of freedom is $G - 1$.

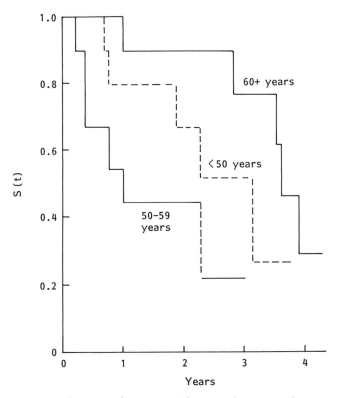

Figure 5.1   Survival curves of women with cervical cancer in three age groups

Table 5.2   Comparison of observed and expected deaths following the first death at 90 days and the general notation used at time t

Time t = 90 Age group	Dead	Alive	Total	$O_{Y,90}$	$O_{M,90}$	$O_{S,90}$	$E_{Y,90}$	$E_{M,90}$	$E_{S,90}$
Young	0	10	10	0	1	0	0.333333	0.300000	0.366667
Middle	1	8	9						
Senior	0	11	11						
Total	1	29	30						

Time t Age group	Dead	Alive	Total	O_{Yt}	O_{Mt}	O_{St}	E_{Yt}	E_{Mt}	E_{St}
Young	a_t	d_t	m_t	a_t	b_t	c_t	$r_t m_t/N_t$	$r_t n_t/N_t$	$r_t l_t/N_t$
Middle	b_t	e_t	n_t						
Senior	c_t	f_t	l_t						
Total	r_t	s_t	N_t						

Table 5.3   Calculation of logrank test for a three-group comparison

Patient number	Rank	Survival (days) Y	M	S		Dead	Alive	Total	E_Y	E_M	E_S
11	1		90		Y	0	10	10	0.333333	0.300000	0.366667
					M	1	8	9			
					S	0	11	11			
						1	29	30			
15	2		142		Y	0	10	10	0.344828	0.275862	0.379310
					M	1	7	8			
					S	0	11	11			
						1	28	29			
23	3		150		Y	0	10	10	0.357143	0.250000	0.392857
					M	1	6	7			
					S	0	11	11			
						1	27	28			
29	4	269			Y	1	9	10	0.370370	0.222222	0.407407
					M	0	6	6			
					S	0	11	11			
						1	26	27			
28	5	272			Y	1	8	9	0.346154	0.230769	0.423077
					M	0	6	6			
					S	0	11	11			
						1	25	26			
6	6		291		Y	0	8	8	0.320000	0.240000	0.440000
					M	1	5	6			
					S	0	11	11			
						1	25	26			
25	7		362		Y	0	8	8	0.333333	0.208333	0.458333
					M	1	4	5			
					S	0	11	11			
						1	23	24			
16	8			373	Y	0	8	8	0.347826	0.173913	0.478261
					M	0	4	4			
					S	1	10	11			
						1	22	23			
27	9		383+								
30	10	468+									
7	11	519+									
18	12		563+								
22	13		650+								
5	14	680			Y	1	5	6	0.352941	0.117647	0.529412
					M	0	2	2			
					S	0	9	9			
						1	16	17			

Table 5.3 (*continued*)

Patient number	Rank	Y	M	S		Dead	Alive	Total	E_Y	E_M	E_S
3	15	827			Y	1	4	5	0.312500	0.125000	0.562500
					M	0	2	2			
					S	0	9	9			
						1	15	16			
24	16		837		Y	0	4	4	0.266667	0.133333	0.600000
					M	1	1	2			
					S	0	9	9			
						1	14	15			
26	17		890+								
13	18			919+							
21	19			978+							
2	20			1037	Y	0	3	3	0.272727	0.090909	0.636364
M	0		1	1							
					S	1	6	7			
						1	10	11			
14	21		1090+								
8	22			1100+							
19	23	1113+									
20	24	1153			Y	1	1	2	0.285714	0.000000	0.714286
					M	0	0	0			
					S	0	5	5			
						1	6	7			
17	25			1297	Y	0	1	1	0.166667	0.000000	0.833333
					M	0	0	0			
					S	1	4	5			
						1	5	6			
10	26			1307	Y	0	1	1	0.200000	0.000000	0.800000
					M	0	0	0			
					S	1	3	4			
						1	4	5			
12	27	1360+									
4	28			1429	Y	0	0	0	0.000000	0.000000	1.000000
					M	0	0	0			
					S	1	2	3			
						1	2	3			
1	29			1476+							
9	30			1577+							

Totals						$E_Y = 4.610203$		$E_M = 2.367988$		$E_S = 9.021806$	
						$O_Y = 5$		$O_M = 6$		$O_S = 5$	
						$n_Y = 10$		$n_M = 9$		$n_S = 11$	

Example

Substituting the values from Table 5.3 in equation (5.1) gives $\chi^2_{\text{Logrank}} = 7.40$. In this example there are $G = 3$ age groups so we have $df = 2$. Reference to Table T3 with $df = 2$ and $\chi^2_{\text{Logrank}} = 7.40$ gives $p = 0.025$. This suggests some evidence of survival difference between the three age groups.

In general, for a contingency table with R rows and C columns, the degrees of freedom is given by $(R-1)(C-1)$. In the above analysis, we are analysing a series of 3×2 contingency tables therefore $R = G = 3$ and $C = 2$ from which we obtain $df = 2$. Such a χ^2 test is termed a test for homogeneity between groups. Using this test we can conclude, for example, that there appears to be larger differences between the three age groups than would be expected by chance alone. However, this test does not identify where the differences occur. This information may be sought in an informal way from Figure 5.1 in this example, or by making further statistical tests using features of the study design.

Example from the literature

Mufti *et al.* (1985) compare patients with myelodysplastic syndromes with respect to three Bournemouth score groupings (0 or 1, 2 or 3, 4) representing the severity of the disease and determined from characteristics at diagnosis. They give $\chi^2_{\text{Logrank}} = 37.96$, $df = 2$ and a p-value $= 0.000001$, demonstrating differences in survival in these three groups.

5.3   TEST FOR LINEAR TREND

As we have indicated earlier, in patients diagnosed with colon cancer, their subsequent survival time is influenced by stage of disease at diagnosis. Thus, experience tells us that a patient with Dukes' A disease is likely to survive longer than a patient with Dukes' B disease. In turn, a patient with Dukes' B disease is likely to survive longer than one with Dukes' C disease. There is, therefore, a natural ordering of the groups which we can make use of in a test for linear trend. Such a test addresses the specific question of whether prognosis deteriorates with stage, rather than the more general question addressed by the test for homogeneity of whether there are any differences in survival between stages.

This test for trend is evolved from the test for trend in a general $G \times 2$ contingency table. Details are given in Altman (1991, sections 10.8.2 and 13.4.3), who points out that the method is equivalent to a regression analysis.

Example

At the beginning of the trial of 30 women with cervical cancer, it may have been suggested that older women have a poorer prognosis than younger women. At the end of the trial a test for a trend in prognosis with age may help us assess the evidence for this hypothesis.

To illustrate the test for trend, consider the last part of Table 5.3, which is extended in Table 5.4. Here the $G(=3)$ age groups are labelled with the value of the variable h_g representing age. In this example, $h_Y = 45$, $h_M = 55$ and $h_S = 65$ years, where 45, 55 and 65 represent the centres of the three age groups of the 30 women. Alternatively, these can be labelled 0, 1 and 2 merely by subtracting 45 and dividing each by 10. Such a change in the code for the h's will usually simplify the arithmetic in what follows. Even more saving on the subsequent arithmetic can be made by further subtracting 1 to obtain the codes $-1, 0, 1$.

The test for trend involving G groups requires the calculation of the following terms:

$$D_g = h_g d_g = h_g (O_g - E_g)$$
$$F_g = h_g E_g$$

and

$$H_g = h_g^2 E_g \tag{5.3}$$

for each group.

These terms are then summed over the G groups to obtain D, F and H. Similarly, we sum E, which is equivalent to the total number of deaths across all groups. The test for trend is then given by

$$\chi^2_{Trend} = D^2/V_{Trend} \tag{5.4}$$

where

$$V_{Trend} = H - (F^2/E). \tag{5.5}$$

This test is a usual χ^2 test, but has $df = 1$ irrespective of the number of groups G.

We emphasise that one should not test for trend after first inspecting the data (see Figure 5.1) as such 'data snooping' exercises may discourage a formal test of the original (design) hypothesis and encourage the substitution of a data-dependent hypothesis to test in its place. For example, in our problem, after the results are in we may postulate that the disease is likely to be more aggressive during the menopausal stage (the intermediate age group) and we may suggest that it is this, rather than age, which is of major prognostic importance.

Table 5.4 Notation for a test for trend

Age group	Age (years)	Coded age	Coded age	h_g	Deaths O_g	E_g	Difference $d_g = O_g - E_g$
Young	45	1	−1	h_Y	O_Y	E_Y	$O_Y - E_Y$
Middle	55	2	0	h_M	O_M	E_M	$O_M - E_M$
Senior	65	3	1	h_S	O_S	E_S	$O_S - E_S$

Table 5.5 Illustration of the calculation of the test for linear trend for the 30 women with cervical cancer

Age group (code, h_g)	Deaths		d_g	D_g	F_g	H_g
	O_g	E_g				
45(−1)	5	4.610	0.390	−0.390	−4.610	4.610
55 (0)	6	2.368	3.632	0.000	0.000	0.000
65 (1)	5	9.022	−4.022	−4.022	9.022	9.022
Total		E = 16.000		D = −4.412	F = 4.412	H = 13.632

Example

The calculations for the 30 women with cervical cancer, classified into three age groups, and using the codes −1, 0 and 1, are summarised in Table 5.5. From this table we obtain

$$V_{Linear} = 13.632 - [(4.412)^2/16.000]$$
$$= 12.415$$

and the test for linear trend gives

$$\chi^2_{Linear} = (-4.412)^2/12.415$$
$$= 1.57.$$

Reference to Table T3 with df = 1 indicates a p-value >0.1. However, since df = 1, a more precise p-value can be obtained by referring $\sqrt{1.57} = 1.25$ to Table T1, which gives a p-value = 0.2113 or 0.21. Thus, a test for linear trend is not statistically significant, as might have been anticipated by inspection of Figure 5.1, since this suggests that the younger women have an intermediate prognosis. We should note that we are using the data here for 'statistical' illustration and not drawing conclusions about relative prognosis in patients with cervical cancer.

In this example, we have replaced 'Trend' in equations (5.4) and (5.5) by 'Linear' as shorthand for 'Linear Trend'. The linear part arises from the specific example because we have used equal age differences between the groups.

Example from the literature

The World Health Organization Task Force on Long-acting Systemic-Agents for Fertility Regulation (1990) investigated the pregnancy rates associated with the differing body weights of women using a contraceptive vaginal ring. Their results are summarised in Table 5.6. These data give $V_{Linear} = 89.81 - (-12.38)^2/26.00 = 83.92$ and $\chi^2_{Linear} = (24.38)^2/83.92 = 7.08$. Reference to Table T3 with df = 1 or Table T1 gives a p-value = 0.008.

This suggests a strong linear effect of increasing pregnancy rate with weight at first use of the ring. The 12-month discontinuation rates for the four weight groups in increasing order are given as 1.8%, 2.6%, 5.3% and 8.2%, respectively, by WHO (1990).

Table 5.6 Observed and expected numbers of pregnancies by weight of women at first use of a vaginal ring (From WHO, Task force on long-acting systemic agents for fertility regulation, 1990. Reproduced by permission of *Lancet* 336: 955–9.)

Weight (kg)	h_g	Number of women (n_g)	Number of pregnancies		$O_g - E_g$	D_g	F_g	H_g
			Observed (O_g)	Expected (E_g)				
−49	−3	227	3	5.28	−2.28	6.84	−15.84	47.52
50–59	−1	425	7	11.33	−4.33	4.33	−11.33	11.33
60–69	1	253	10	6.72	3.28	3.28	6.72	6.75
70+	3	100	6	2.69	3.31	9.93	8.07	24.21
Total		1005	26	E = 26.00		D = 24.38	F = −12.38	H = 89.81

There is no requirement in the test for trend that the codes (sometimes referred to as weights), h_g, have to be equally spaced. For example, if the Senior women of Table 5.1 were better represented by an age group centred at 70 (rather than 65), then h_S may be set at 70. This would result in codes of either 2.5, or 1.5, depending on which code for body weight is used in the calculation. A different value for χ^2_{Trend} will result, but this is a consequence of the change in the codes and would be expected.

5.4 NON-LINEAR TREND

In the preceding section, we have referred to linear trend since, for example, with the 30 women with cervical cancer we were assuming a linear change in prognosis with age as displayed by the use of the codes −1, 0, and 1. Suppose, however, we had postulated at the beginning of the trial that the menopausal women (the middle age group) might have the worst prognosis. In this situation, one can test for non-linear (quadratic) trend by assigning codes h_g equal to 1, −2, and 1 to the successive age groups. The calculations proceed using equations (5.3), (5.4) and (5.5) but with the new values for h_g.

Example

If we apply the weights 1, −2, 1 to the data of Table 5.5 we obtain E = 16.000 as before, but D = −10.896, F = 8.896 and H = 23.104. Therefore

$$V_{Quadratic} = 23.104 - [(8.896)^2/16.000]$$
$$= 18.1578.$$

The test for quadratic trend gives

$$\chi^2_{Quadratic} = (-10.896)^2/18.1578$$
$$= 6.54.$$

Reference to Table T3 with df = 1 indicates a p-value <0.02. More precise calculations, using Table T1, give a p-value = 0.0105 or 0.01. Thus, a test for quadratic trend indicates, from this illustrative data set, that there is some evidence that menopausal women have poorer survival.

5.5   FACTORIAL DESIGNS

The basic reason for using a factorial design in a clinical trial is that two (or more) types of treatment may be compared simultaneously. Conventionally, the types of treatment are termed **factors** and the alternatives within each factor the **levels**. A 2×2 factorial design will have two factors **A** and **B**. Each factor has two levels, a first and a second level, denoted **(1)** and **a** for Factor **A** and **(1)** and **b** for Factor **B**. The two factors are combined to give four (2×2) treatment combinations **(1)(1)**, **a(1)**, **(1)b** and **ab**, which are conventionally summarised by **(1)**, **a**, **b** and **ab** respectively. The **(1)** represents the combination treatment of the first level of Factor **A** with the first level of Factor **B**. Combination treatment **a** represents the second level of Factor **A** with the first level of Factor **B**. Combination treatment **b** represents the first level of Factor **A** with the second level of Factor **B**. Finally, combination treatment **ab** represents the second level of Factor **A** with the second level of Factor **B**. We note that in practice the first level of a factor will often mean the absence of that factor.

Example

As an example, Factor **R** may represent postoperative (adjuvant) radiotherapy for patients with a certain cancer and Factor **C** adjuvant chemotherapy. A randomised clinical trial to assess the value of radiotherapy and/or chemotherapy in this setting could well have a factorial design since it may be that neither therapy helps to improve survival. In this case **(1)** represents the no radiotherapy and no chemotherapy option, **r** the radiotherapy without chemotherapy option, **c** the chemotherapy without radiotherapy option and **rc** the combined modality option of both radiotherapy and chemotherapy. Patients eligible for this trial would be randomised to one of the four treatment options.

Example from the literature

Nash *et al.* (1990) describe a randomised trial of two levels of frequency, **F**, and two types of stimulation, **S**, with transcutaneous nerve stimulation (TENS) to relieve pain in patients with chronic pain. The two levels of Factor **F** are a low frequency of 10 Hz and a high frequency of 100 Hz. The two levels of Factor **S** are non-continuous (pulse) stimulation and a continuous stimulation. In the notation introduced above the four treatment options are therefore **(1)** = low frequency and pulse stimulation, **f** = high frequency and pulse stimulation, **s** = low frequency and continuous stimulation and **fs** = high frequency and continuous stimulation. The investigators recruited 50 patients to each of the four options of the 2×2 design. Their results are summarised in Figure 5.2, which suggests that those patients

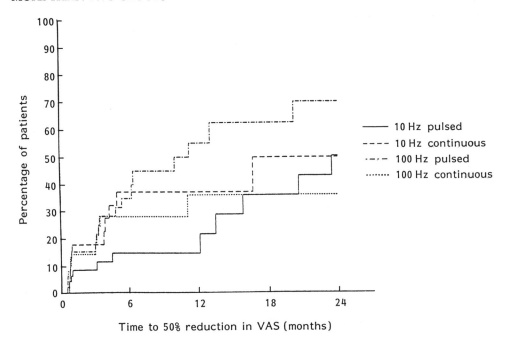

Figure 5.2 Kaplan–Meier estimate of the cumulative percentage of patients achieving a 50% reduction in visual analogue score (VAS) from baseline values for four types of TENS (From Nash *et al.*, 1990. Reproduced by permission of VSP International Science Publishers.)

receiving high-frequency (100 Hz), pulse stimulation TENS treatment may experience the greater benefit.

In the analysis of a 2×2 factorial design to estimate the main effect of Factor **A**, patients who receive **ab** are compared with those who receive **b**, and patients who receive **a** are compared with those who receive (**1**). We use the shorthand, main effect of Factor **A**, to represent the difference in effect of the two levels of Factor **A**. The mean of these two comparisons is then taken to obtain a main effect of Factor **A**. This process is expressed as

$$[\mathbf{A}] = \frac{\{[\mathbf{ab}] - [\mathbf{b}]\} + \{[\mathbf{a}] - [\mathbf{1}]\}}{2}. \tag{5.6}$$

Here the brackets, [.], denote the 'statistical measure' from those patients receiving the particular treatment option. For survival time studies, such a measure will be the corresponding $O - E$ for that particular group. From equation (5.6), we can see that the main effect of Factor **A** is obtained by taking an average of two effects: the effect of **A** at the second level of Factor **B** and the effect of **A** at the first level of Factor **B**.

In a similar way, the main effect of Factor **B** is

$$[\mathbf{B}] = \frac{\{[\mathbf{ab}] - [\mathbf{a}]\} + \{[\mathbf{b}] - [\mathbf{1}]\}}{2}. \tag{5.7}$$

Example from the literature

Table 5.7 summarises the results of the randomised trial, conducted by Nash *et al.* (1990), in which 55 of 200 patients experienced reduction in their pain levels during the course of treatment and follow-up. It is worth emphasising (see chapter 10, which is concerned with sample sizes, for details) that although 200 patients have been recruited to this trial the number of events observed is only 55 (27.5%). Consequently, the trial does not have high statistical power for the question(s) intended.

The values of $d = (O - E)$ corresponding to the four treatment groups are given in Table 5.7. Combined in the format of equation (5.6), these give the main effect for high versus low frequency treatment as

$$[F] = \frac{\{[fs] - [s]\} + \{[f] - [1]\}}{2}$$

$$= \frac{\{(12 - 12.8) - (13 - 11.4)\} + \{(19 - 13.5) - (11 - 17.3)\}}{2}$$

$$= \frac{\{-0.8 - 1.6\} + \{5.5 + 6.3\}}{2}$$

$$= 9.4/2 = 4.7.$$

This suggests that the high-frequency TENS achieves more remissions than the low-frequency TENS, since $[F] = 4.7$ is positive.

In more familiar terms, this can be alternatively expressed as a hazard ratio (HR). This is obtained by summing the observed and expected values for pulse and continuous in Table 5.7 for each frequency. This gives for 10 Hz, $O_{10} = 11 + 13 = 24$, $E_{10} = 17.3 + 11.4 = 28.7$ and for 100 Hz $O_{100} = 19 + 12 = 31$, $E_{100} = 13.5 + 12.8 = 26.3$. Finally $HR_F = (31/26.3)/(24/28.7) = 1.41$, suggesting a benefit to the high-frequency TENS.

A formal test of significance for the main effect of frequency is a stratified logrank test of the form described in equation (4.16). This takes the form of comparing the groups **fs** with **s** and **f** with **(1)**. It is calculated as

$$\chi_F^2 = (24 - 28.7)^2/28.7 + (31 - 26.3)^2/26.3$$

$$= (4.7)^2\left(\frac{1}{28.7} + \frac{1}{26.3}\right)$$

$$= 1.61.$$

Table 5.7 Observed and expected numbers of patients who achieved 50% reduction in pain levels (From Nash *et al.*, 1990. Reproduced by permission of VSP International Science Publishers.)

			Number of patients achieving pain relief			
Frequency (Hz)	Stimulation	Number of patients	Observed (O)	Expected (E)	Difference (O − E)	Ratio O/E
10	Pulse (1)	50	11	17.3	−6.3	0.63
	Continuous (s)	50	13	11.4	1.6	1.14
100	Pulse (f)	50	19	13.5	5.5	1.41
	Continuous (fs)	50	12	12.8	−0.8	0.94

This result is far from statistically significant since use of Table T1 with $z = \sqrt{1.61} = 1.27$ gives a p-value $= 0.2041$. It is useful to note that $[F] = 4.7$ appears in the numerator of the expression for χ_F^2.

In a similar way, the main effect of the type of stimulation is

$$[S] = \frac{\{[fs] - [f]\} + \{[s] - [1]\}}{2}$$

$$= \frac{\{(12 - 12.8) - (19 - 13.5)\} + \{(13 - 11.4) - (11 - 17.3)\}}{2}$$

$$= \frac{\{-0.8 - 5.5\} + \{1.6 + 6.3\}}{2}$$

$$= 1.6/2 = 0.8.$$

This suggests that continuous-stimulation TENS achieves more remissions than pulsed TENS. However, the magnitude of this effect is less than that of using high- as opposed to low-frequency TENS. The corresponding HR calculated in a similar way to HR_F is $HR_S = (25/24.2)/(30/30.8) = 1.06$ suggests a marginal benefit to the continuous as opposed to pulse stimulation.

A stratified logrank test with df $= 1$ gives $\chi_S^2 = (30 - 30.8)^2/30.8 + (25 - 24.2)^2/24.2 = 0.05$. This is again far from statistically significant since use of Table T1 with $z = \sqrt{0.05} = 0.22$ gives a p-value $= 0.8259$.

There is one other important comparison that can be assessed in a factorial design and that is the interaction effect. This is estimated by

$$[AB] = \{[ab] - [a] - [b] + [1]\}/2 \tag{5.8}$$

and should be compared with equations (5.6) and (5.7). The interaction effect is aimed at assessing whether the effect of Factor (treatment) **A** is similar at the two levels of Factor **B**. Similarly, because of the symmetry in expression (5.8) between **A** and **B**, it also assesses whether the effect of **B** is similar at the two levels of Factor **A**. If there is good evidence of an interaction, i.e. the effect of **A** appears to be different at the lower and higher levels of Factor **B**, then taking the simple average effect, as given in equation (5.6), to be the estimate of the effect of Factor **A** may be questioned. Emphasis may be placed on the individual effects at the higher and lower levels of Factor **B**, depending on practical considerations. By symmetry, similar considerations hold for Factor **B**.

Example

For the data of Table 5.6 we have

$$[FS] = \{[fs] - [f] - [s] + [1]\}/2$$
$$= \{(12 - 12.8) - (19 - 13.5) - (13 - 11.4) + (11 - 17.3)\}/2$$
$$= \{0.8 - 5.5 - 1.6 - 6.3\}/2$$
$$= -14.2/2 = -7.1.$$

In this example, the interaction effect $[FS]$ is larger than either of the main effects $[F]$ or $[S]$. This can be seen from Table 5.6 in that the effect, for example, of pulsed stimulation with 100 Hz is to increase the relief rate $(O/E = 1.41)$, but has the opposite effect with 10 Hz (O/E = 0.63). We note that this differential effect can only be estimated if a factorial design is used for the trial.

The relevant HR for summarising the interaction is $HR_{FS} = (23/30.1)/(32/24.9) = 0.59$ where $23 = 11 + 12$, $30.1 = 17.3 + 12.8$, $32 = 13 + 19$ and $24.9 = 11.4 + 13.5$, from Table 5.7. This suggests that it is better giving either low-frequency continuous or high-frequency pulsed as opposed to either low-frequency pulsed or high-frequency continuous TENS. However, some care needs to be taken in drawing such a conclusion from these data, as the number of events observed is small and, therefore, associated CIs will be wide.

A formal logrank test for the [FS] interaction with df = 1 gives $\chi^2_{FS} = (23 - 30.1)^2/30.1 + (32 - 24.9)^2/24.9 = 3.70$. This is larger than the corresponding values for the main effects and leads, from Table T1, with $z = \sqrt{3.70} = 1.92$, to a p-value = 0.0549. We note, however, that the test for interaction will only generally be sensitive enough to detect relatively large interaction effects. The associated Kaplan–Meier curves for the Factor F and Factor S comparisons are shown in the panels of Figure 5.3.

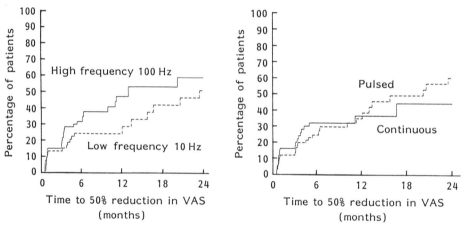

Figure 5.3 Kaplan–Meier estimate of the percentage of patients achieving a 50% reduction in VAS from baseline values for low and high frequency and for pulse and continuous frequency types of TENS (From Nash *et al.*, 1990. Reproduced by permission of VSP International Science Publishers.)

Example from the literature

The cumulative risk of myocardial infarction (MI) and death in the first 30 days during treatment as reported by The RISC Group (1990) is shown in Figure 5.4. The four treatment groups used in this trial were in a 2×2 factorial form. This figure suggests a benefit of aspirin and an apparent lack of benefit of heparin either given alone or as an addition to aspirin treatment.

When analysing 2×2 factorial designs in which the data are *not* of the survival type, it can be shown that the χ^2_A, χ^2_B and the χ^2_{AB} each with df = 1 sum to the overall χ^2 test for homogeneity with df = G – 1 = 3. For technical reasons, associated with

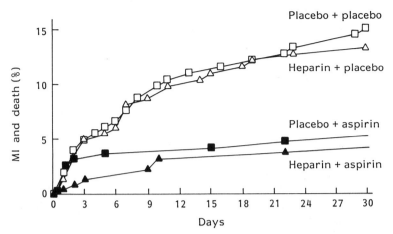

Figure 5.4 Risk of myocardial infarction (MI) and death during treatment with aspirin, heparin, both and none (From the RISC Group, Risk of myocardial infarction and death during treatment with low dose aspirin and intravenous heparin in men with unstable coronary artery disease. *Lancet*, 336, 827–830, © by The Lancet, 1990)

summing over tables at different death times t, together with the different numbers of events occurring in each treatment, this is not generally true for survival data. It is usually best to analyse factorial designs using a Cox regression model as described in chapter 6. This approach avoids technical difficulties that can occur.

5.6   THE MANTEL–HAENSZEL TEST

We noted in section 4.5 that the logrank test can be modified to become the Mantel–Haenszel test by a change in the method of estimating the variance V (compare equations (4.4) and (4.11)). Similar considerations apply to the G (>2) group situation, although the procedure and the calculations become more complex. Such calculations are, in fact, best left to standard computer packages. However, we illustrate the procedure for the G = 3 situation and extend it by analogy to more than three groups.

The formal calculation of the Mantel–Haenszel test in the two-group situation, equation (4.11), can be expressed in the following way:

$$\chi^2_{MH} = d^2/V = dV^{-1}d \qquad (5.9)$$

where $d = (O - E)$ can be taken for either one of the groups A or B, $V = \Sigma\, m_t n_t r_t s_t / [N_t^2(N_t - 1)]$ and V^{-1} is the inverse of V or $1/V$. We will see the justification for the last (rather clumsy) format of equation (5.9) by the analogy with equation (5.19) below.

The reason that only one of A or B appears in this expression is because of the symmetry. In particular the variance does not change if we substitute A for B in equation (4.11) since they are both equal magnitude and only differ in sign

$(d_B = -d_A)$, and so their squared values are equal.

$$Var(a_t) = Var(b_t) = m_t n_t r_t s_t / [N_t^2(N_t - 1)]. \tag{5.10}$$

This expression is given in Table 4.4.

In addition to these two variances, there is also the covariance of a_t with b_t. This is

$$Cov(a_t, b_t) = -m_t n_t r_t s_t / [N_t^2(N_t - 1)] \tag{5.11}$$

and has been referred to in equation (4.25).

The negative sign arises in equation (5.11) as a consequence of the fact that if we increase (decrease) a_t by unity in our 2×2 table at time t, but keep the same marginal totals m_t, n_t, r_t, s_t, then b_t must decrease (increase) to compensate. This necessary change in the value of b_t indicates a negative correlation between a_t and b_t. In fact, this covariance term does not appear in the expression (5.9) for the two-group situation. However, for the case of $G = 3$ (or more) groups, A, B and C, we need the variances and covariances of (any) pair of a_t, b_t and c_t as there are 2 df for a 3×2 contingency table. In practice, this is because if we change a_t by unity, but retain the same marginal totals m_t, n_t, l_t, r_t and s_t of Table 5.2, we now have the choice of compensating for this change with either b_t or c_t.

Using the notation of Table 5.2 we have

$$Var(a_t) = m_t(n_t + l_t)r_t s_t / [N_t^2(N_t - 1)] \tag{5.12}$$

for a three-group situation. To obtain this expression we first combine the cells of Table 5.2 corresponding to B and C which sum to $(n_t + l_t)$. This then replaces n_t in equation (5.10) and is the only change required. Similarly, combining A and C gives

$$Var(b_t) = n_t(m_t + l_t)r_t s_t / [N_t^2(N_t - 1)]. \tag{5.13}$$

Finally, combining A and B we have

$$Var(c_t) = l_t(m_t + n_t)r_t s_t / [N_t^2(N_t - 1)]. \tag{5.14}$$

The covariance term, $Cov(a_t, b_t)$ remains as (5.11) while

$$Cov(b_t, c_t) = -n_t l_t r_t s_t [N_t^2(N_t - 1)] \tag{5.15}$$

and there is a similar expression for $Cov(a_t, c_t)$.

To obtain the corresponding total (summed) variances and covariances the terms are added together, one for each table at event time t. Remember that at times when no deaths occur, there is no corresponding table. For brevity, we label these totals Var(A), Var(B), Var(C), Cov(A,B), Cov(B,C) and Cov(A,C). It should be remembered that $Cov(x,y) = Cov(y,x)$ in all circumstances.

However, the Mantel–Haenszel test only requires the values for any two of the groups. We choose A and B for convenience. We write them in the following (matrix) format:

$$\mathbf{V} = \begin{bmatrix} Var(A) & Cov(A, B) \\ Cov(B, A) & Var(B) \end{bmatrix}. \tag{5.16}$$

This matrix has two rows and two columns. We now require a matrix for the corresponding two differences $d_A = O_A - E_A$ and $d_B = O_B - E_B$. We can write this either as a single-column matrix, with two rows and one column:

$$d = \begin{bmatrix} d_A \\ d_B \end{bmatrix} \qquad (5.17)$$

or alternatively as a single-row matrix, with one row and two columns:

$$d' = [d_A, d_B]. \qquad (5.18)$$

The rules of matrix multiplication require that we need both of the d and d' forms. Finally, we write, in a very compact form, the Mantel–Haenszel test statistic as

$$\chi^2_{MH} = d'V^{-1}d. \qquad (5.19)$$

This can be compared with equation (5.9) above. This expression is often used to describe the test in the general case of G groups. In this case, d will have one column of $G - 1$ terms, while V and V^{-1} (the latter is termed the inverse of the matrix V) will be $(G - 1) \times (G - 1)$ square matrices.

To do the formal calculation for the Mantel–Haenszel test, it is first necessary to obtain V^{-1} from equation (5.16). In mathematical terms we need to invert the matrix V. In the 2×2 case it can be shown that the inverse matrix is

$$V^{-1} = \begin{bmatrix} \text{Var}(B)/M & -\text{Cov}(A,B)/M \\ -\text{Cov}(A,B)/M & \text{Var}(A)/M \end{bmatrix} \qquad (5.20)$$

where $M = \text{Var}(A)\text{Var}(B) - [-\text{Cov}(A,B)]^2$.

To evaluate equation (5.19), we first calculate $V^{-1}d$, which is equivalent to multiplying the individual terms in the first row of the matrix V^{-1} by the corresponding terms in the column of matrix d and summing, then doing the same with the second row of V^{-1}. This gives

$$V^{-1}d = \begin{bmatrix} [d_A \text{Var}(B) - d_B \text{Cov}(A,B)]/M \\ [-d_A \text{Cov}(A,B) + d_B \text{Var}(A)]/M \end{bmatrix}.$$

This matrix has only a single column with two elements. These elements are then multiplied by the corresponding elements of the row matrix d and summed to obtain finally

$$\begin{aligned} \chi^2_{MH} &= d'V^{-1}d \\ &= [d_A^2 \text{Var}(B) - d_A d_B \text{Cov}(A,B) - d_B d_A \text{Cov}(A,B) + d_B^2 \text{Var}(A)]/M \\ &= [d_A^2 \text{Var}(B) - 2d_A d_B \text{Cov}(A,B) + d_B^2 \text{Var}(A)]/M. \qquad (5.21) \end{aligned}$$

The corresponding expressions for $G > 3$ groups become very complex indeed. Fortunately they are not usually required since numerical values calculated from the data are placed in V rather than the general algebraic expressions. There are sophisticated, accurate and fast ways of inverting matrices and these are used in the corresponding statistical computer packages when required.

On occasions, and usually in the more mathematical statistical texts, equation (5.19) is written as

$$\chi^2_{MH} = d'V^-d \qquad (5.22)$$

Here there is a minor change to the exponent of V in that the 1 is omitted. This is done to restore the symmetry to the expression by including all G treatment groups when describing $\mathbf{V}$. Thus, for $G = 3$, we have

$$\mathbf{V} = \begin{bmatrix} \text{Var}(A) & \text{Cov}(A, B) & \text{Cov}(A, C) \\ \text{Cov}(B, A) & \text{Var}(B) & \text{Cov}(B, C) \\ \text{Cov}(C, A) & \text{Cov}(C, B) & \text{Var}(C) \end{bmatrix}. \tag{5.23}$$

This shows the full make-up of the study design.

The matrix $\mathbf{V}^-$ is termed the *generalised inverse* rather than the *inverse* of $\mathbf{V}$, which is the $\mathbf{V}^{-1}$. In a similar way, we have modified $\mathbf{d}'$ to include all treatment groups. Thus, for $G = 3$, we have

$$\mathbf{d}' = [d_A, d_B, d_C] \tag{5.24}$$

and there is a parallel expression for $\mathbf{d}$.

6 Cox's Proportional Hazards Model

Summary

This chapter introduces Cox's proportional hazards model, which is used extensively in the analysis of survival data. The use of the model includes assessing treatment effects in studies and in particular adjusting these comparisons for baseline characteristics. A comparison of the method of calculating hazard ratios (HRs) with that derived following the logrank test of chapter 4 is made. A further use of these models is to assess variables for prognostic significance. In this context the use of both continuous and categorical variables in a model is described.

6.1 INTRODUCTION

We have described in earlier chapters the concept of the hazard rate, or the instantaneous event rate. If the distribution of survival times can be assumed exponential, then this rate is estimated by the ratio of the number of events observed divided by the total survival time, as given in equation (3.4). One consequence of the assumption of the exponential distribution of survival time is that the hazard rate, λ, does not vary with time. For example, in a clinical trial, this would imply that the underlying death rate in the first year of patient follow-up equals the death rate in each subsequent year. One example where this would not apply is if there is an excess mortality in the immediate postsurgical period, say 30 days, in patients undergoing leg amputation. This may be because of possible complications from infection. Thereafter the risk of death is known to be smaller. We express this possible lack of a constant value by noting that the hazard rate may depend on follow-up time, t, and we therefore write $\lambda(t)$ in place of λ to reflect this.

A guide to whether or not the hazard rate can be regarded as constant is to plot the complementary log transformation, which is $\log\{-\log[S(t)]\}$, against $\log t$, as we have illustrated in Figure 3.4. If the hazard rate does not change with time then the resulting plot will be approximately linear. Departures from linearity indicate that the hazard rate is changing with time. For reasons of brevity we often refer to the hazard rather than more correctly to the hazard rate.

Example

The complementary log plots of two groups of patients with non-small cell lung cancer (NSCLC) are shown in Figure 6.1. One group consists of those patients who presented with NSCLC but without evidence of metastatic disease; the other group is made up of patients in which metastatic disease was detected. These data are taken from two randomised trials of the Medical Research Council Lung Cancer Working Party (1991, 1992) and comprise the 304 patients who received the same course of radiotherapy (F2) which was a treatment common to each trial. This aspect of these trials has been discussed in more detail by Wheeler *et al.* (1994).

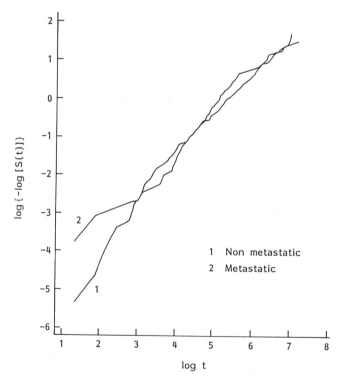

Figure 6.1 Graph of $\log\{-\log[S(t)]\}$ against $\log t$ in patients treated with radiotherapy with metastatic and non-metastatic non-small cell lung cancer (data from Medical Research Council Lung Cancer Working Party, 1991, 1992, reproduced by permission of The Macmillan Press Ltd)

The plots of the hazards for the two groups in Figure 6.1 are approximately linear and overlapping. This suggests that not only is the hazard constant within each group but also that it is similar for both patient groups.

Example

Figure 6.2 shows the complementary log plots for two groups of patients with small cell lung cancer (SCLC). These patients all received a combination chemotherapy of etoposide, cyclophosphamide, methotrexate and vincristine (ECMV) for their disease. This was the common treatment arm used in three randomised trials of the Medical Research Council Lung Cancer Working Party (1989a, 1989b, 1993). In total 932 patients presented at diagnosis with either limited or extensive SCLC and were randomised to receive ECMV. This aspect of these trials has again been discussed in more detail by Wheeler *et al.* (1994).

In contrast to the patient groups with NSCLC illustrated in Figure 6.1, the hazard in both the limited and extensive disease groups appears to vary with time since the two graphs are non-linear. Nevertheless, the two plots appear 'parallel' in that there is an approximately constant vertical distance between them at any given time. In this situation we say that the hazards for the two patient groups are proportional,

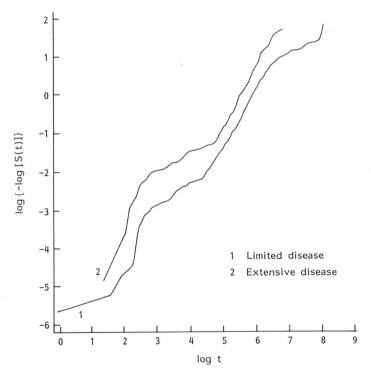

Figure 6.2 Graph of log {−log[S(t)]} against log t in patients treated with ECMV chemotherapy with limited and extensive small cell lung cancer (data from Medical Research Council Lung Cancer Working Party, 1989a, 1989b, 1993, reproduced by permission of The Macmillan Press Ltd)

i.e. their ratio remains approximately constant with time. For the patients with NSCLC of Figure 6.1, this ratio is approximately 1, because the lines are approximately coincident.

The purpose of this chapter is to relate non-constant hazards, $\lambda(t)$, to variables which may influence their value. Such variables are often those recorded at presentation of the patient for diagnosis or at the time of entry into a study. They may include variables describing the nature of the disease, demographic characteristics of the patient and the treatment received.

6.2 PROPORTIONAL HAZARDS

In investigating a group of patients with cancer of the brain, we might wish to relate the length of their survival to various clinical characteristics that they have at diagnosis, for example tumour grade, history of fits, age and treatment received. To do this, it is first useful to define an underlying hazard for the 'average' patient with brain cancer. We denote this average hazard by $\lambda_0(t)$. We can then specify the hazard for a particular patient, $\lambda(t)$, in relation to this average hazard by

$$\lambda(t) = h(t)\lambda_0(t) \tag{6.1}$$

where $h(t)$ is a function which may change with time t. That is, we describe the hazard $\lambda(t)$ of a particular patient as a multiple, $h(t)$, of the average hazard, $\lambda_0(t)$. We can rewrite equation (6.1) as a ratio of the particular patient hazard to the average hazard. This gives the so-called relative hazard as

$$h(t) = \frac{\lambda(t)}{\lambda_0(t)}. \tag{6.2}$$

If $h(t)$ does not change with time then we write $h(t) = h$, where h is a constant. Consequently, we can write h in place of $h(t)$ in equation (6.1), since the relative hazard no longer depends on t.

Example

We have noted from Figure 6.2 that for any time t the ratio of the hazards for groups of patients with extensive and limited disease SCLC is approximately constant, although the individual hazards appear to change with time.

Note, however, even when both $\lambda(t)$ and $\lambda_0(t)$ change with time their ratio can remain constant. In this situation, we say the hazards are proportional. This implies that at any given time t the hazard rate applying to our particular patient will be h times that of the average patient with this disease.

In situations where $h(t) = 1$, for all values of t, then the hazard rate $\lambda(t)$, at a given time t, for any particular patient, does not differ from the average of $\lambda_0(t)$.

Example

The metastatic and non-metastatic patients with NSCLC of Figure 6.1 have approximately the same hazard. In this case the relative hazard of equation (6.2) is $h(t) = h = 1$.

We have seen in chapter 3, when discussing the exponential and Weibull distributions, that the logarithm of the hazard is often used. As a consequence it is convenient to write $h(t) = e^{\beta(t)} = \exp[\beta(t)]$. This implies $\beta(t) = \log h(t)$, so that when the hazards are proportional equation (6.2) can be written as

$$\log[h(t)] = \log h = \log\left[\frac{\lambda(t)}{\lambda_0(t)}\right] = \beta. \qquad (6.3)$$

The strength of the proportional hazards model developed by Cox (1972), which we now describe, is not only that it allows a non-constant hazard rate to be modelled, but it does so without making any assumption about the underlying distribution of the hazards in different groups, except that the hazards in the groups remain proportional over time.

6.3 COMPARING TWO TREATMENTS

Suppose we have patients with brain tumours randomised to receive one of two therapies, standard (control, C) or test (new, N), and we wish to determine whether treatment N improves patient survival.

We write the hazard for those receiving C as

$$\lambda_C(t) = \lambda_0(t). \qquad (6.4)$$

This assumes that all patients receiving C have the same underlying hazard $\lambda_0(t)$. If we then assume that the hazards are proportional for patients in the two treatment groups, we can write the hazard for those receiving N as

$$\lambda_N(t) = \lambda_0(t)\exp(\beta). \qquad (6.5)$$

This is equivalent to saying that the hazard for patients receiving N is a constant, here $\exp(\beta)$, times that of the patients who receive C. The hazard rate (HR) for patients receiving the respective treatments is the ratio of the hazards given by equations (6.5) and (6.4), respectively. Thus

$$HR = \frac{\lambda_N(t)}{\lambda_C(t)} = \frac{\lambda_0(t)\exp(\beta)}{\lambda_0(t)} \qquad (6.6)$$

or

$$HR = \exp(\beta). \qquad (6.7)$$

The influence of time on the hazard is summarised in $\lambda_0(t)$ and this is divided out in equation (6.6). As a consequence, the HR is a constant since equation (6.7) does not depend on t. It follows from equation (6.7) that $\log HR = \beta$.

Example

To illustrate the estimation of β, we use the data from patients with brain cancer who were recruited to a randomised trial of the Medical Research Council Working

Party on Misonidazole in Gliomas (1983). The patients were treated either by radiotherapy alone (C) or by radiotherapy with the radiosensitiser misondidazole (N). A total of 198 patients received C and 204 received N. For illustration, a portion of the data set are given in Table 6.1.

Using the BMDP (1988) statistical package gives, for the full data set, the estimate of β for equation (6.7) as b = −0.0563, from which HR = e^b = exp(−0.0563) = 0.9452. Such an HR implies a better risk for patients receiving the new therapy since HR < 1 and equation (6.6) then implies $\lambda_N(t) < \lambda_C(t)$.

In addition to the estimate b of β, the BMDP computer output provides the associated standard error, SE(b). The test of the null hypothesis of no difference between the control and new treatments is equivalent to testing the hypothesis that $\beta = 0$ in equation (6.7). This in turn is equivalent to testing HR = 1 since, in this case,

Table 6.1 Survival time and some baseline characteristics for 30 patients with brain cancer receiving radiotherapy alone or radiotherapy plus the sensitiser misonidazole (Part data from Medical Research Council Working Party on Misonidazole in Gliomas, 1983. Reproduced by permission of The British Institute of Radiology.)

Patient number	Received misonidazole	Fits before entry	Tumour grade	Age (years)	Survival time (days)	Survival status
1	NO	NO	4	48	1084	ALIVE
2	YES	NO	3	63	22	DEAD
3	YES	NO	4	54	40	DEAD
4	NO	NO	3/4	49	25	DEAD
5	YES	NO	4	44	487	DEAD
6	NO	YES	4	36	696	DEAD
7	YES	NO	3	29	887	ALIVE
8	NO	NO	3	50	336	DEAD
9	NO	NO	4	53	213	ALIVE
10	NO	YES	3	58	361	DEAD
11	YES	NO	3	48	244	DEAD
12	YES	NO	4	49	799	DEAD
13	YES	NO	3/4	60	180	DEAD
14	NO	YES	3	49	488	DEAD
15	NO	NO	4	64	121	DEAD
16	YES	YES	4	61	210	DEAD
17	NO	YES	3	41	575	ALIVE
18	NO	NO	4	58	258	DEAD
19	YES	NO	4	35	273	DEAD
20	YES	NO	3	42	1098	ALIVE
21	YES	YES	3/4	30	819	ALIVE
22	YES	NO	3	66	14	DEAD
23	NO	YES	3	48	734	DEAD
24	YES	YES	4	57	225	DEAD
25	NO	NO	3/4	56	152	DEAD
26	YES	YES	3	43	207	DEAD
27	YES	YES	3	33	943	ALIVE
28	NO	NO	3	39	581	DEAD
29	YES	YES	3/4	48	371	DEAD
30	NO	NO	3	55	85	ALIVE

HR $= \exp(\beta) = e^0 = 1$. One method of testing this hypothesis is to calculate the z-statistic of equation (1.10) which, in this case, is

$$z = b/SE(b). \tag{6.8}$$

We then refer z to Table T1 of the standard Normal distribution to obtain the p-value. Alternatively

$$W = z^2 = [b/SE(b)]^2 \tag{6.9}$$

can be referred to Table T3 of the χ^2 distribution with degrees of freedom (df) equal to 1. In this format the test is termed the Wald test and is discussed further in section 6.14.

Example

The computer output for the trial of therapies for patients with brain cancer gave $b = -0.0563$ and $SE(b) = 0.1001$. Thus, use of equation (6.8) gives $z = -0.0563/0.1001 = -0.56$. Referring $z = 0.56$ to Table T1 gives a p-value $= 0.5755$. With such a large p-value we would not reject the null hypothesis of equal efficacy of treatments C and N.

In most contexts, it is often appropriate to calculate a confidence interval (CI) rather than merely rely on a test of statistical significance alone. By analogy with equation (4.6) the $100(1 - a)\%$ CI for log HR is given by

$$b - z_{1-a/2}SE(b) \qquad \text{to} \qquad b + z_{1-a/2}SE(b). \tag{6.10}$$

The $100(1 - a)\%$ CI for the population HR is, therefore, given by analogy with equation (4.7) by

$$\exp[b - z_{1-a/2}SE(b)] \qquad \text{to} \qquad \exp[b + z_{1-a/2}SE(b)]. \tag{6.11}$$

Example

For the patients with brain cancer we have $b = -0.0563$, and $SE(b) = 0.1001$. The corresponding 95% CI is calculated by setting $a = 0.05$ in equation (6.10) to obtain $z_{0.975} = 1.96$ from Table T2 and hence $\exp[-0.0563 - (1.96 \times 0.1001)] = 0.78$ to $\exp[-0.0563 + (1.96 \times 0.1001)] = 1.15$. This 95% CI contains the null hypothesis value, HR $= 1$ (or equivalently $\beta = 0$), of no treatment difference. Nevertheless there still remains some uncertainty about the true efficacy of the treatments as expressed by the HR. For example, both an HR $= 0.8$ indicating benefit to N and HR $= 1.1$ suggesting an adverse benefit of N are not inconsistent with the 95% CI obtained.

6.4   THE COX MODEL

In fact, we can combine both equations (6.4) and (6.5) into a single expression, by introducing the indicator variable x for treatment received, and writing

$$\lambda(t) = \lambda_0(t) \exp(\beta x). \tag{6.12}$$

If the patient receives control therapy, C, then we set $x = 0$ and the right-hand side of equation (6.12) becomes that of equation (6.4), since $\beta x = 0$ and $e^0 = 1$. If the patient receives the new treatment, N, then $x = 1$ and the right-hand side becomes equation (6.5), since $\beta x = \beta$.

Finally, we can write equation (6.12) even more compactly, as

$$\mathbf{T} : h_x = \exp(\beta x) \tag{6.13}$$

where $x = 0$ or 1 depending on the treatment group. Thus $h_0 = 1$, $h_1 = \exp(\beta)$ and, when comparing the two treatment groups, $HR = h_1/h_0 = \exp(\beta)$ also.

This expression again emphasises that in proportional hazard circumstances the HR does not depend on t. In this format equation (6.13) is termed the Cox proportional hazards model. Thus variable x helps to describe or model the variation in the relative hazard. The variable x is often referred to as the regressor variable and β as the regression coefficient or parameter.

We use the notation $\mathbf{T}$ here to denote the model which is examining the influence of treatment. The null hypothesis of no treatment difference is expressed as $\beta = 0$ in (6.13), in which case $HR = h_1/h_0 = 1$. When using the Cox proportional hazards model we estimate the parameter β from the data.

Example

The estimate of $HR = 0.9452$ in the above calculation, using the Cox model for the full brain cancer patient data corresponding to Table 6.1, is very close to the estimate given by the use of equation (4.5), following the logrank test. In our example, this gives $HR_{Logrank} = (O_N/E_N)/(O_C/E_C) = (204/209.61)/(198/193.39) = 0.9456$. The expected number of deaths, E_C and E_N, are obtained from output provided by BMDP. This estimate differs from the Cox estimate only in the final figure, due to rounding errors in the two procedures. The corresponding Mantel–Haenszel estimate from equation (4.12) is $HR_{MH} = \exp[(O_N - E_N)/V] = \exp\{(204 - 209.61)/88.75\} = 0.9387$, which is close to these estimates. The value of V is also obtained from output provided by BMDP.

In fact, when including only one variable, here x, the Cox proportional hazards approach with the use of the score test (see section 6.14) and the Mantel–Haenszel form of the logrank test are identical. This equivalence means that when treatment comparisons are performed the Mantel–Haenszel form of the logrank test is more widely used because of its simplicity and relative ease of understanding.

6.5 BINARY VARIABLES

One important problem is to identify the potential prognostic importance of binary (Yes or No) variables: for example, whether individuals, having had no experience of fits before diagnosis, have a different survival than patients with brain cancer type who have experienced fits (F). For this purpose, we can use the same formulation for the Cox model as for when comparing two treatments. In this case, the equivalent expression to equation (6.13) is

$$F: h_{x_F} = \exp(\beta_F x_F) \qquad (6.14)$$

where $x_F = 0$ if the patient has had no fits before diagnosis and $x_F = 1$ if the patient has experienced fits. We denote the model as F and the regression parameter to be estimated is β_F. We ignore the possible influence of other variables here. We can write the hazard ratio (HR_F) as the ratio of the relative hazard in those who have experienced a fit compared to the relative hazard in those that have not. Thus

$$HR_F = \frac{h_1}{h_0}$$

$$= \exp(\beta_F).$$

Example

For the patients with brain cancer, BMDP gives the estimate of $b_F = -0.3925$ with $SE(b_F) = 0.1159$. This gives an estimate of $HR_F = \exp(b_F) = \exp(-0.3925) = 0.6754$. This is less than 1, indicating, perhaps somewhat counterintuitively, that patients with a history of fits have a better prognosis than those who have not. The clinical explanation for this is that a history of fits in the patient tends to suggest that the brain tumour has been present for some time and is slow growing and, therefore, not so aggressive. This contrasts with tumours in patients with no such history and which, therefore, may be rapidly growing and hence bring a poor prognosis.

As before, the null hypothesis of no difference between the two groups is considered by testing whether $\beta_F = 0$. A formal test of this null hypothesis using equation (6.8) gives, $z = b_F/SE(b_F) = 3.3877$, which from Table T1 gives a p-value = 0.0007. Thus there is strong evidence that the parameter $\beta_F \neq 0$ and that a previous history of fits does imply improved survival.

Example from the literature

Mayo *et al.* (1991) use the Cox proportional hazards model to investigate factors influencing recovery time from stroke to full and independent sitting function in 45 post-stroke victims who were not self-sitting immediately following their stroke. One factor they considered that was likely to influence patient recovery was the degree of perceptual impairment, which they categorised in binary form as none-to-mild or moderate-to-severe. They observed a HR = 0.26 with a 95% CI of 0.10 to 0.66 and concluded from this that those with the least degree of perceptual impairment recovered more quickly. This HR corresponds to $b = -1.35$ and $SE(b) = 0.48$, giving $z = -1.35/0.48 = -2.8$ and p-value = 0.005. This confirms the influence of the degree of perceptual impairment on recovery time.

6.6 CONTINUOUS VARIABLES

We have indicated that one advantage of the proportional hazards model over the logrank test is that it can be used with continuous variables. We illustrate this use to assess the importance of actual age (rather than, for example, age group as used in Table 5.2) in the prognosis of patients with brain cancer (Table 6.1). For the purpose of this example we ignore the possible influence of a history of fits, tumour grade and treatment received, on survival in these patients. By analogy with equations (6.13) and (6.14) we can specify the Cox model taking account of age as

$$A : h_{Age} = \exp(\beta_A A) \tag{6.15}$$

where A is the age of the patient and β_A is the corresponding regression coefficient.

Example

If this model is fitted to the brain cancer data, then $b_A = 0.0320$ and $SE(b_A) = 0.0049$. We note that $HR = \exp(b_A) = \exp(0.0320) = 1.033$. The corresponding test statistic is $z = 0.0320/0.0049 = 6.53$ with an associated p-value <0.001, obtained by reference to Table T2, which indicates for $z = 3.2905$ that the p-value $= 0.0010$. Clearly $z = 6.53$ is larger than this and, therefore, implies a p-value <0.001. More comprehensive tables of the Normal distribution give a p-value <0.0000001. This suggests that age is a very clear predictor of survival.

If we wish to compare the survival experience of two patients, of ages A_1 and A_2 respectively, then, from (6.15), we have

$$h_{Age\,1} = \exp(\beta_A A_1)$$

and

$$h_{Age\,2} = \exp(\beta_A A_2).$$

The ratio of these is

$$HR = \frac{h_{Age\,1}}{h_{Age\,2}} = \frac{\exp(\beta_A A_1)}{\exp(\beta_A A_2)} = \exp[\beta_A(A_1 - A_2)]. \tag{6.16}$$

Thus, the HR depends only on the difference in age, $(A_1 - A_2)$, of the two patients under consideration.

Example

A patient aged 50 (A_1), compared to one aged 40 (A_2), will have an estimated hazard ratio $HR = \exp[b_A(50 - 40)] = \exp(0.0320 \times 10) = 1.3771$. This suggests very strongly that the older patient has the much greater risk of death once diagnosed with this disease. Since the patients differ in age by 10 years we note that $1.033^{10} = 1.3771$.

For technical reasons it is quite usual, in the case of continuous variables, to write the Cox model (6.15) with age expressed as a difference from the mean age of the patients under consideration. Thus, we write the relative hazard as

$$A:h_{Age} = \exp[\beta_A(A - \bar{A})] \qquad (6.17)$$

where $\bar{A}$ is the mean age of the patients. A quick check with $A_1 - \bar{A}$ and $A_2 - \bar{A}$ replacing A_1 and A_2 in equation (6.16) shows that this change does not affect the final estimate of the HR for the two patients since $(A_1 - \bar{A}) - (A_2 - \bar{A}) = A_1 - A_2$.

Example

For the brain cancer analysis above, the mean age of the patients is $\bar{A} = 52.3$ years and $b_A = 0.0320$; thus the model described by equation (6.17) is

$$A:h_{Age} = \exp[0.0320(Age - 52.3)].$$

This model can be written as

$$h_{Age} = \exp(0.0320\,Age) \times \exp[0.0320 \times (-52.3)]$$

or

$$h_{Age} = 0.1876\,\exp(0.0320\,Age).$$

For an individual of age 40, i.e. 12.3 years below the mean

$$h_{40} = 0.1876\,\exp(0.0320 \times 40) = 0.1876\,\exp(1.28)$$
$$= 0.6747$$

This calculation gives the same results as setting $b_A = 0.0320$ in place of β_A, $A_1 = 40$ and $A_2 = 52.3$ directly in equation (6.16).

Similarly, for a patient aged 50, we have $h_{50} = 0.1876\,\exp(0.0320 \times 50) = 0.1876$ $\exp(1.60) = 0.9292$. Finally this gives HR $= h_{50}/h_{40} = 0.9292/0.6747 = 1.3772$. This is the value we had obtained previously for the HR except for rounding error in the fourth decimal place.

Using the form of the Cox model presented in equation (6.17), we can now state that an individual of average age has $h_{Age} = 1$, since for this patient $(A - \bar{A}) = 0$. We can now also see that since the estimate of $b_A = 0.0320$ is positive, that individuals below the mean age have a decreased hazard. This is because $(A - \bar{A})$ is negative for such a patient, hence $b_A(A - \bar{A})$ is negative and exponentiating a negative quantity gives a HR < 1. For individuals whose age is above the mean of the group the hazard is increased. Here $(A - \bar{A})$ is positive, hence $b_A(A - \bar{A})$ is also positive and exponentiating a positive quantity gives a HR > 1.

6.7 TWO EXPLANATORY VARIABLES

As already indicated, it is well known in patients with brain cancer that a history of fits prior to diagnosis is of prognostic importance. In fact having had previous fits may be more of a determinant of patient survival than the form of treatment given. In such a situation, where more than one variable may influence survival, we can extend the Cox proportional hazards model. To assess the influence (if any) of both treatment and history of fits, we combine equations (6.13) and (6.14) into one model containing two variables, as

$$\mathbf{T} + \mathbf{F} : h = \exp(\beta_T x_T + \beta_F x_F). \tag{6.18}$$

Here x_T refers to treatment and x_F to a history of fits and β_T, β_F are the corresponding regression coefficients. The x's are coded as $x_T = 0$ for standard treatment (radiotherapy alone, C) and $x_T = 1$ for test treatment (radiotherapy plus misonidazole, N). Similarly $x_F = 0$ if the patient has had no history of fits, and $x_F = 1$ if the patient has previously experienced fits. We should note that model (6.18) for $\mathbf{T} + \mathbf{F}$ is merely the product of equations (6.13) and (6.14), which are the models for $\mathbf{T}$ and $\mathbf{F}$, respectively.

Alternatively, equation (6.18) can be expressed as

$$\log h = \beta_T x_T + \beta_F x_F. \tag{6.19}$$

Using this model, there are now four groups of patients. For those who receive radiotherapy alone (control) and have had no history of fits ($x_T = 0$, $x_F = 0$) and that $h = \exp(0) = 1$. This implies that the hazard for this particular group (control treatment who have had no history of fits) is equal to the underlying hazard, $\lambda_0(t)$. We therefore regard this as the baseline group against which we compare the other patient groups.

For expository purposes here, we introduce the notation $h_{x_T x_F}$ for the hazard to indicate that its value may change according to treatment received ($\mathbf{T}$), ($x_T = 0$ or 1), and history of fits ($\mathbf{F}$), ($x_F = 0$ or 1). Thus, $h_{00} = 1$ represents the hazard for the 'baseline' group. The choice of which group to be used as the baseline is arbitrary and usually depends on which is most convenient in the context of the example being considered. Those patients who receive the new therapy and have had no history of fits have ($x_T = 1$, $x_F = 0$), giving $h_{10} = \exp(\beta_T)$. Those who receive the control treatment but have experienced fits have ($x_T = 0$, $x_F = 1$) with $h_{01} = \exp(\beta_F)$ and finally those who receive the new therapy and who also have experienced fits have ($x_T = 1$, $x_F = 1$), with $h_{11} = \exp(\beta_T + \beta_F)$.

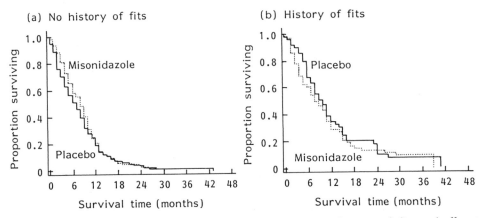

Figure 6.3 Survival in patients with brain cancer by prior history of fits and allocated treatment group (From Medical Research Council Working Party on Misonidazole in Gliomas, 1983. Reproduced by permission of The British Institute of Radiology.)

It is worth noting that, the ratios

$$\frac{h_{11}}{h_{01}} = \frac{\exp(\beta_T + \beta_F)}{\exp(\beta_F)} = \exp(\beta_T + \beta_F - \beta_F) = \exp(\beta_T) = HR_T$$

and

$$\frac{h_{10}}{h_{00}} = \frac{\exp(\beta_T)}{\exp(0)} \qquad = \exp(\beta_T - 0) \qquad = \exp(\beta_T) = HR_T.$$

Both have the same value, which is the HR for the treatment comparison. This implies that the treatment effect, which is measured by the size of β_T, is assumed to be the same, both for patients who have had a history of fits prior to diagnosis and for those patients who have had no such history.
Similarly,

$$\frac{h_{11}}{h_{10}} = \frac{\exp(\beta_T + \beta_F)}{\exp(\beta_T)} = \exp(\beta_F) = HR_F$$

and

$$\frac{h_{01}}{h_{00}} = \frac{\exp(\beta_F)}{\exp(0)} \qquad = \exp(\beta_F) = HR_F.$$

These imply that with this model the effect on survival of having or not having a history of fits is the same, irrespective of the treatment received.

Example

The Kaplan–Meier estimates of the survival curves of the four treatment by history of fits groups of patients with brain tumours are shown in Figure 6.3 (a, b). They are given in two panels to aid clarity of presentation as there is some overlap in the curves in the early months following randomisation. Figure 6.3(a), which shows the survival curves by treatment group for those patients with no history of fits, suggests, if anything, a slight advantage to those receiving misonidazole. In contrast, Figure 6.3(b), which shows the survival curves by treatment group for those patients with a history of fits, suggests, if anything, a slight disadvantage to those receiving misonidazole. If this indeed was the case then the assumption that this treatment effect, β_T, is constant in both groups of patients would not hold.
It is possible, however, to check if this is indeed the case by extending the Cox model to include an interaction term as discussed later in section 6.11. For this trial, the analysis (see Table 6.2) suggests the absence of any real difference between treatments. This means that the small differences indicated by Figures 6.3 (a, b) are likely to be random. The Cox model of equation (6.18) fitted to these data gives the regression coefficients summarised in Table 6.2. The estimate $b_T = -0.0486$ for the treatment comparison, with corresponding $HR_T = \exp(-0.0486) = 0.9526$. This is only very slightly changed from $b = -0.0563$ with corresponding $HR_T = \exp(-0.0563) = 0.9452$, given earlier. The latter was derived from the Cox model for T without information on fits included. Such a small change may not always occur,

Table 6.2 Cox proportional hazards model fitted to history of fits and treatment of the patients with brain cancer (From Medical Research Council Working Party on Misonidazole in Gliomas, 1983. Reproduced by permission of The British Institute of Radiology.)

Variable	Coefficient	Estimate (b)	$HR = e^b$	SE(b)	b/SE(b)	p-value
Treatment	β_T	−0.0486	0.9526	0.1001	−0.4854	0.6274
History of fits	β_F	−0.3913	0.6762	0.1159	−3.3767	0.0007

for example, if the proportions of patients having a history of 'fits' and 'no fits' differed markedly in the two treatment groups. If by chance one of the treatments is given to substantially more patients of good prognosis then it may, as a consequence, appear to be the better treatment, since good-prognosis patients survive longer in any event.

For the presence of history of fits, the $HR_F = \exp(-0.3913) = 0.6762$. This represents a substantially reduced risk of death in those who have experienced fits as compared to those who have not. For history of fits, $z = -0.3913/0.1159 = -3.38$ and use of Table T1 gives a p-value <0.002. This suggests, as we have already observed, that patients with a history of fits do indeed have a better prognosis than those with no history of fits. More extensive tables of the Normal distribution give the p-value $= 0.0007$.

The statistical 'significance' of the regression coefficients in a Cox model is discussed further in section 6.14 and chapter 7.

6.8   MORE THAN TWO EXPLANATORY VARIABLES

The Cox model can be extended to include more than two variables. Thus, the influence of age (x_A) on the survival of patients with brain cancer could be added to the model describing the effect of treatment (x_T) and history of fits (x_F). In this case the relative hazard for the extended model is

$$\mathbf{T} + \mathbf{F} + \mathbf{A} : h = \exp(\beta_T x_T + \beta_F x_F + \beta_A x_A). \tag{6.20}$$

Here x_A is a continuous variable whilst x_T and x_F are binary. To ease presentation and description we have written x_A rather than $(x_A - \bar{x}_A)$ here although we have used the latter in actual calculations.

Example

Fitting the three-variable model of equation (6.20) to the data from the patients with brain cancer gives the results summarised in Table 6.3. This shows that both history of fits and age, even when both are included in the same model, appear to influence survival, although there are smaller values for both the treatment and history of fits regression coefficients, as compared to those of Table 6.2.

Table 6.3 Cox's model incorporating treatment, stage and age in 417 brain cancer patients (From Medical Research Council Working Party on Misonidazole in Gliomas, 1983. Reproduced by permission of The British Institute of Radiology.)

Variable	Coefficient	Estimate (b)	HR = e^b	SE(b)	b/SE(b)	p-value
Treatment	β_T	−0.0326	0.9680	0.1001	−0.3251	0.7451
Fits	β_F	−0.2729	0.7612	0.1169	−2.3339	0.0196
Age	β_A	0.0303	1.0308	0.0049	6.1395	<0.0001

The number of variables that can be added to the Cox model is, in theory, without end. Thus, in general, we have a v-variable regression model for the relative hazard, of the form

$$h = \exp(\beta_1 x_1 + \beta_2 x_2 + \dots + \beta_v x_v). \tag{6.21}$$

Now although the number of variables we can add is without limit, there are practical constraints since estimates have to be obtained for the regression coefficients. Thus, for example, we cannot include more variables in a model than subjects available for the analysis. One 'rule of thumb' is not to include more variables than the fourth root of the number of events available for analysis. For the brain cancer trial of our example there are 417 patients, with 402 deaths having been observed. This suggests that we should not include more than $402^{1/4} = 4.47$ or approximately four variables in a Cox model. With four variables in the model, each will have at least two possible values (treating age here as either young or old for brevity), implying $2^4 = 16$ categories. With 402 deaths, this suggests an average of $402/16 = 25$ deaths per category group. A second 'rule of thumb', therefore, suggests we should have a reasonable number of subjects in each subcategory of interest before constructing a regression model.

Another 'rule of thumb' is to have at least 15–20 events for every additional variable that we are including in the model. This rule suggests that rather more than four variables may be appropriate for investigation with the brain data. Simon and Altman (1994) give a comprehensive discussion of these issues.

Example from the literature

Meng *et al.* (1988) investigated factors influencing the recovery of sperm production following cessation of gossypol treatment in 46 Chinese males. The factors considered were serum follicle-stimulating hormone (FSH), serum luteinising hormone (LH), serum testosterone, total acid phosphatase, age, weight, duration of gossypol treatment and testicular volume. Their final model includes three variables: duration of gossypol treatment (G), corrected testicular volume (V) and FSH (F). Since both duration of gossypol treatment and FSH have rather skew distributions a log scale was chosen for these variables. The model is

$$G + V + F : \log h = -0.313 \text{ [log duration of gossypol (years)} - 1.15]$$
$$+ 0.075 \text{ [corrected testicular volume (ml)} - 29.1]$$
$$- 0.0578 \text{ [log FSH (IU/ml)} - 1.73].$$

They fit three variables to data in which only 28 events (recovery of sperm production) are observed. Such a limited number of events would suggest that there is likely to be considerable uncertainty in the values of the regression coefficients reported. In this model all three prognostic variables are continuous and are treated as such. We note that each variable is expressed relative to the mean in the format of equation (6.17).

6.9   CATEGORICAL VARIABLES

We have discussed earlier how to include a binary variable, such as treatment group or history of fits, into the Cox model. Suppose, however, that we are concerned with assessing the influence of tumour grade (see Table 6.1). There are three tumour grade groups: those patients of definitely Grade 3, those of definitely Grade 4 and an intermediate group of Grade 3/4. In such cases, we ask the basic question as to whether or not tumour grade is influential on prognosis.

   One way of doing this is to fit a Cox model using so-called dummy variables to describe the variable Grade. We first create, in our case two, dummy variables as follows:

$$g_1 = 1 \text{ intermediate Grade 3/4 patient}$$
$$g_1 = 0 \text{ not an intermediate Grade 3/4 patient}$$
$$g_2 = 1 \text{ Grade 4 patient}$$
$$g_2 = 0 \text{ not a Grade 4 patient}$$

In this way the three grade groups correspond to different pairs of values of (g_1, g_2) in the following way. The pair, $g_1 = 0$ and $g_2 = 0$, define Grade 3 patients since the values of g indicate neither an intermediate Grade 3/4 patient nor a Grade 4 patient. Similarly, the pair, $g_1 = 1$ and $g_2 = 0$, define intermediate Grade 3/4 patients and finally the pair, $g_1 = 0$ and $g_2 = 1$, define Grade 4 patients.

   The Cox model for Grade, ignoring all other potential variables, is then written as

$$G : \log h = \gamma_1 g_1 + \gamma_2 g_2. \tag{6.22}$$

This model can then be fitted to the data in the same way as earlier models.

   In this model there are two regression coefficients, γ_1 and γ_2, to estimate. These are both concerned with grade. In general, if a categorical variable has g categories then $g - 1$ dummy variables need to be created for the corresponding terms in a Cox model and consequently $g - 1$ regression coefficients have to be estimated.

Example from the literature

A Cox regression model reported by Fisher *et al.* (1991) was used to assess the relative influence of 11 potential prognostic variables in 914 patients with breast cancer. The authors reduce the number of variables to the five shown in Table 6.4 by rejecting those variables for which the associated χ^2, analogous to equation (6.9), gave a test statistic yielding a p-value > 0.2. Each of the remaining variables—age,

Table 6.4 Cox model to determine predictors of time to development of distant disease in patients with breast cancer (From Fisher *et al.*, 1991, Significance of ipsilateral breast tumour recurrence after lumpectomy, *Lancet*, 338, 327–331, © by The Lancet Ltd)

Variable	b	SE(b)	χ^2	p	HR	95% CI
Age (years)						
<50	0	–			1	
≥50	0.268	0.113	5.77	0.016	1.31	1.05–1.63
Nodal status						
Negative	0	–			1	
Positive	0.402	0.111	12.99	0.0003	1.49	1.20–1.86
Nuclear grade						
Good	0	–			1	
Poor	0.405	0.117	11.98	0.0005	1.50	1.19–1.89
Tumour type						
Good	0	–			1	
Intermediate	0.492	0.217	5.75	0.017	1.64	1.07–2.50
Poor	0.758	0.224	13.33	0.0003	2.13	1.38–3.31
Maximum pathological tumour size						
<2 cm	0	–			1	
≥2 cm	0.274	0.111	6.06	0.014	1.32	1.06–1.63

nodal status, nuclear grade, tumour type and tumour size—had a p-value < 0.2, in fact < 0.02. As a consequence, the HRs quoted for these variables have associated 95% CIs which do not include HR = 1.

If we focus on the analysis of tumour type in Table 6.4 and ignore the remainder of the table, then the results are summarised in Table 6.5. The model for the corresponding relative hazard is therefore

$$\mathbf{TT} : \log h = 0.492\, g_1 + 0.758\, g_2.$$

Thus, when the tumour type is Good, $g_1 = g_2 = 0$, $\log h = 0$ and this provides the baseline group. Similarly, when the tumour type is Intermediate, $g_1 = 1$, $g_2 = 0$ and $\log h = 0.492$. Finally, when the tumour type is Poor, $g_1 = 0$, $g_2 = 1$ and $\log h = 0.758$. The corresponding HRs, expressed as relative to Good tumour type are therefore, $\exp(0.492) = 1.64$ and $\exp(0.758) = 2.13$ for Intermediate and Poor tumour types, respectively.

Table 6.5 Cox model assessing the influence of tumour type on time to development of distant metastases in patients with breast cancer (part of Table 6.4)

Tumour type (TT)	Dummy variable, g_1	Dummy variable, g_2	Regression coefficient, (b)	SE(b)	HR
Good	0	0	0	–	1
Intermediate	1	0	0.492	0.217	1.64
Poor	0	1	0.758	0.224	2.13

In many circumstances, the categorical variables can be placed on a numeric scale. Suppose, for example, since the categories of tumour type (Good, Intermediate, Poor) are clearly ordered, they are included in a Cox model with the single associated variable g taking values 0, 1 and 2. This approach assumes a linear trend in prognosis as tumour type changes, since biological differences between tumour types have been given equal numerical steps of unity. Such an approach is equivalent to describing the change in regression coefficients in Table 6.5 by the broken line in Figure 6.4. Here the relationship is summarised by one regression coefficient which is the slope of the line. If a linear relationship can be assumed then this model provides a very powerful test of this trend. The final model, however, is of the same form as equation (6.15) which is for a continuous variable. Thus, a numerically ordered categorical variable is treated in a similar way to a continuous variable in the modelling process.

A question often arises as to whether a continuous variable should or should not be transformed into a categorical variable for analysis. For example, is it better to 'categorise' the variable age into three separate categories say, less than 50 (Young), 50–59 (Middle Aged) and 60 or more (Senior), as we did in section 5.3, or to leave it as a continuous variable in a Cox model?

The answer often lies in the use to be made of the prognostic factor and on the prior information available. If prior information tells us that the prognosis

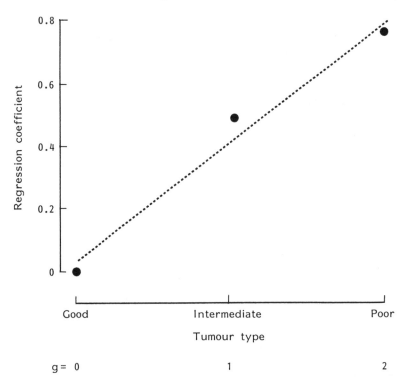

Figure 6.4 Linear relationship between tumour type and time to development of distant metastases in patients with breast cancer (data taken from Table 6.4)

gradually changes with increasing age and we want to know how important a prognostic factor age is, then we may want to employ it as a continuous variable. In doing this, we are assuming that age is approximately linearly related to prognosis. If, however, age is acting, say, as a surrogate for menopausal status in women with a particular disease, then categories of −44, 45–54, 55+ may then be thought of as 'definitely' premenopausal, perimenopausal and 'definitely' postmenopausal. In such circumstances, it is this categorisation that is thought to be more important than age itself.

If we are not sure, for example, of the relationship between the variable age and survival, or want to use the prognostic factor 'age' in practice, then transforming the variable into categories may be advisable. It is then appropriate to include age as a series of dummy variables, and to use the equivalent of equation (6.22) with age (Young, Middle Aged, Senior) in place of Tumour Type (Good, Intermediate, Poor) of Table 6.5.

In making a continuous variable discrete, a number of decisions have to be made. First, we must decide how categories should be made. Although this depends on the context, we recommend no more than four categories and that three is usually sufficient. Secondly, the boundaries for these categories need to be considered carefully. These should be derived in such a way as to make divisions at numerically simple values, ensure sufficient numbers in each category and, most importantly, make clinical sense. For example, the age divisions described above are centred about the mean age of 52.3 years using the category Middle Aged for those patients aged 45 to 54 inclusive, with numerically convenient boundaries. As already indicated, this division makes biological sense. A final check of the data should verify that sufficient patients, of the order of 25%, say, are included in each group. Often it it is useful to choose boundaries that are the same as those used by others working in a similar context, since we might wish to make comparisons with these related studies.

6.10 THE ANALYSIS OF A 2 × 2 FACTORIAL STUDY

In randomised control clinical trials it is possible, in appropriate circumstances, to pose two or more treatment questions simultaneously. For example, in the AXIS trial (Gray et al., 1991), which is enrolling patients with colorectal cancer, there are two basic questions. One is the value of radiotherapy, and the second the value of postoperative hepatic infusion of fluorouracil, in prolonging survival in these patients. In brief, there are four treatments corresponding to the two factors: infusion (**I**) and radiotherapy (**R**). The use of (**1**), **I**, **R** and **I** + **R** notation for models has been introduced in chapter 5. These four treatments are summarised in Table 6.6.

The analysis of such a 2 × 2 factorial design has been described in section 5.5 using the logrank test. An alternative approach is by means of the following Cox model, using an analogy with equations (6.18) and (6.21). Using the notation introduced in section 6.7, this model is

$$\mathbf{I} * \mathbf{R} : h_{x_I x_R} = \exp(\beta_I x_I + \beta_R x_R + \beta_{IR} x_I x_R). \tag{6.23}$$

Table 6.6 Models for a 2×2 factorial design of the AXIS trial (Reproduced from Gray *et al.*, 1991, with permission of The Macmillan Press Ltd)

Treatment options		Model	Dummy Variable	
			x_I	x_R
No radiotherapy and no infusion	(1)	Null	0	0
No radiotherapy but infusion	I	Infusion	1	0
Radiotherapy but no infusion	R	Radiotherapy	0	1
Radiotherapy and infusion	I + R	Infusion and radiotherapy	1	1

Equation (6.23) gives, for the various combinations of values of x_I and x_R of Table 6.6, the following models:

$$\begin{aligned}
\text{Null model (1)} &: h_{00} = 1 \\
\text{Infusion I} &: h_{10} = \exp(\beta_I) \\
\text{Radiotherapy R} &: h_{01} = \exp(\beta_R) \\
\text{I + R + I.R} &: h_{11} = \exp(\beta_I + \beta_R + \beta_{IR}).
\end{aligned} \tag{6.24}$$

The regression coefficient β_{IR} in the **I + R + I.R** part of the model emphasises the possibility of some interaction between the two treatment types in their effect on survival (see section 6.11) when both treatment types are given simultaneously. This would imply that the effect of, say, the infusion would depend on whether or not radiotherapy was given. If no interaction is present then $\beta_{IR} = 0$ and the model reduces to a main effects model only. That is, the two treatments act independently of each other. This model is

$$\mathbf{I + R} : h = \exp(\beta_I + \beta_R). \tag{6.25}$$

We note that the model of equations (6.24) can be written as **I∗R** as we have done in equation (6.23). This is a convenient shorthand often used in statistical texts and computer package manuals.

Example from the literature

In an example previously presented in Figure 5.4, the cumulative risk of myocardial infarction (MI) and death in the first 30 days during treatment is reported by the RISC Group (1990). The four treatment combinations used in the trial were a 2×2 factorial arrangement of placebo (1), aspirin (a), heparin (h) and aspirin with heparin (ah). This figure suggests a benefit of aspirin with a reduction in 30-day morbidity of more than 5% compared to placebo. It also suggests lack of efficacy of heparin given either alone or in combination with aspirin treatment, which implies little evidence of the presence of an interaction between aspirin and heparin, so that a model **A + H** analagous to equation (6.25) is likely to be appropriate.

We discuss the general approach of including and testing an interaction term in a model in section 6.11.

6.11 INTERACTIONS

As is indicated by equation (6.23), the interaction term in a model is obtained by using a regression coefficient, β_{IR}, with a multiplication term involving $x_I x_R$ from the variables concerned. However, the application of equations, like (6.23) above, is not restricted to the analysis of designed experiments involving only two factors with two levels. It can be extended to more complex designs, and also to applications when the variables under consideration do not include a variable for treatment.

Example

It is of some interest to see in the example of patients with brain cancer whether there is any interaction between history of fits (F) and grade of the disease (G). For example, does the influence of grade on prognosis differ between those patients with a history of fits and those without? Here, for simplicity, tumour grade, which is a categorical variable with $g = 3$ values, is now treated as a binary variable with values $x_G = 0$ for both Grade 3 and Grade 3/4 tumours and $x_G = 1$ for Grade 4 tumours. There are now only $g = 2$ categories for grade and, thus, only one regression coefficient to be estimated. The corresponding overall model is

$$F + G + F.G : h = \exp(\beta_F x_F + \beta_G x_G + \beta_{FG} x_F x_G).$$

The results of fitting this model including the interaction term and the main effects model without the interaction term, which essentially assumes $\beta_{FG} = 0$, are summarised in Table 6.7.

It can be seen from Table 6.7 that the regression coefficient for the interaction term, $b_{FG} = -0.0488$, is not large and has an associated $SE(b) = 0.1183$. These give $z = -0.0488/0.1183 = -0.41$ and from Table T1 a p-value $= 0.6818$. This then implies that we have no evidence of an interaction between history of fits and tumour

Table 6.7 Test for interaction between a history of fits and tumour grade in 417 patients with brain cancer (From Medical Research Council Working Party on Misonidazole in Gliomas, 1983. Reproduced by permission of The British Institute of Radiology.).

	Model			
	Main effects only $F + G$		Including interaction term $F + G + F.G$	
Coefficient	Regression coefficient	SE	Regression coefficient	SE
Fits β_F	−0.3924	0.1159	−0.3379	0.1748
Grade β_G	0.0144	0.0518	0.0269	0.0601
Interaction β_{FG}	–	–	−0.0488	0.1183
χ^2	11.69		11.86	

grade. As a consequence, we use the main effects model, i.e. $F + G : h = -0.3924x_F + 0.0144x_G$, to summarise the data.

We should note that omitting the interaction term from the model changes the estimates of the regression coefficients corresponding to β_F and β_G. This is because, while small, $b_{FG} = -0.0488$ does not equal zero, although we suspect the corresponding parameter $\beta_{FG} = 0$.

It is important to emphasise, however, that tests of interaction have little statistical power. The χ^2 values given in the last row of Table 6.7 are discussed in more detail below and in chapter 7. At this stage we note that $\chi^2_{F+G+F.G} - \chi^2_{F+G} = 11.86 - 11.69 = 0.17$ and $\sqrt{0.17} = 0.41$. This corresponds to the $z = -0.41$ that we obtained earlier for the test of the interaction term.

If the interaction term of Table 6.7 had been statistically significant then we would have retained the model $F*G$, which is shorthand for $F + G + F.G$, rather than the main effects only model $F + G$. In such a circumstance the final model is therefore

$$F*G : h = \exp(-0.3379x_F + 0.0269x_G - 0.0488x_Fx_G).$$

The four patient groups are defined by the combinations of x_F and x_G, i.e. $(0,0)$, $(0,1)$, $(1,0)$ and $(1,1)$ respectively. Thus, the relative hazards are $h_{00} = \exp(0) = 1$, which is the baseline relative hazard, $h_{01} = \exp(0.0269) = 1.0272$, $h_{10} = \exp(-0.3379) = 0.7133$ and finally, $h_{11} = \exp(-0.3379 + 0.0269 - 0.0488) = \exp(-0.3598) = 0.6978$. These then give the ratios $h_{11}/h_{10} = 0.6978/0.7133 = 0.9783$, which estimates the effect of tumour grade in those patients without a history of fits. Similarly, $h_{01}/h_{00} = 1.0272/1 = 1.0272$ estimates the effect of tumour grade in those patients with a history of fits.

Just as we noted when discussing Figure 6.3, these two ratios measuring the effect of tumour grade on prognosis are not exactly equal. In the presence of interaction, we would have to interpret the final model with some care. In our example, however, the regression coefficient for the interaction term is very small and so has little effect. Consequently, the two estimates of the HR for grade, 0.9783 and 1.0272, for the no history and history of fits groups respectively, are approximately equal with a value close to 1. Thus, they can be combined into one estimate which is obtained from fitting model $F + G$.

6.12   STRATIFIED ANALYSIS AND THE COX MODEL

It is possible to perform an analysis adjusting a treatment effect for imbalances in important prognostic factors either by using a stratified logrank test (see section 4.6) or by means of a Cox model. As already noted for a single factor the two approaches are 'equivalent' if the Mantel–Haenszel form of the logrank test is used.

It may be argued that the stratified analysis is easier to explain to non-statisticians and thus it is preferable. However, a stratified logrank test cannot deal with continuous variables without categorisation. In addition, if there are many variables that influence prognosis, the logrank approach becomes tedious. However, the stratified test, unlike the Cox model, does not require proportional hazards for the variables.

Whichever procedure is to be used, it is good practice to specify this before the analysis is performed and to report this in any subsequent publication.

Example

For the patients with brain cancer, the format of the stratified logrank test corresponding to the Cox model, summarised in Table 6.2, is shown in Table 6.8. Thus, for example, for the patients receiving control therapy with no history of fits, the observed and expected number of deaths $O_C = 153$, $E_C = 130.07$ and $O_C - E_C = 19.93$. For those who have experienced fits, the corresponding $O_C = 45$, $E_C = 62.32$ and $O_C - E_C = 45 - 62.32 = -17.32$.

The estimate of the stratified logrank HR for the treatment comparison is obtained using equation (4.15) as

$$HR = [(146 + 58)/(137.15 + 72.47)]/[(153 + 45)/(130.07 + 62.32)]$$
$$= (204/209.62)/(198/192.39)$$
$$= 0.9456$$

This is equal to that obtained from the Cox model of Table 6.2 and suggests a marginal benefit of misonidazole as an addition to radiotherapy.

Example from the literature

A total of 443 eligible patients with Grade 3 or 4 malignant glioma were randomised after surgery into an MRC Brain Tumour Working Party trial (Bleehen et al., 1991) comparing 45 Gy radiotherapy given in 20 fractions over 4 weeks, with 60 Gy given in 30 fractions over 6 weeks. Using a 1:2 randomisation in favour of the higher dose, 144 patients were allocated to receive 45 Gy and 299 were allocated

Table 6.8 Logrank survival comparison by history of fits and treatment in patients with brain cancer (From Medical Research Council Working Party on Misonidazole in Gliomas, 1983. Reproduced by permission of The British Institute of Radiology.)

| Treatment | Fits | Number of patients | Number of deaths | | (O/E) | HR |
			Observed (O)	Expected (E)		
Control	No	156	153	130.07	1.18	1
Misonidazole	No	148	146	137.15	1.06	0.8983
Control	Yes	49	45	62.32	0.72	0.6102
Misonidazole	Yes	64	58	72.47	0.80	0.6780
Totals		417	402	402.01		

Table 6.9 Age distribution of patients with brain cancer by treatment allocated (From Medical Research Council Brain Tumour Working Party, Bleehen *et al.* 1991, with permission.)

Age (years)	Percentage of patients allocated treatment	
	45 Gy	60 Gy
18–39	15	16
40–49	24	18
50–59	27	36
60–73	34	30
Total (%)	100	100
Number of patients	144	299

to receive 60 Gy. A standard logrank analysis of the survival data gave $\chi^2_{\text{Logrank}} = 4.06$, df = 1, p-value = 0.04 and a HR = 0.81 in favour of 60 Gy, with a reported 95% CI of 0.66 to 0.99.

However, as the authors of the report point out, this logrank analysis may underestimate the true benefit of the higher dose of radiotherapy because of a chance unfavourable age distribution in the high dose group. The age distributions of patients in the two treatment groups is summarised in Table 6.9.

Although the age distribution does not appear markedly unbalanced, an adjusted analysis was performed, in which age and treatment allocated were included in a Cox proportional hazards model. In this model, age was included as a continuous variable, because it is known that increasing age is associated with poorer prognosis in this disease.

The model led to an HR = 0.75 in favour of 60 Gy and a 95% CI of 0.61 to 0.92 with an associated p-value = 0.007. Thus, this adjusted analysis gave a somewhat larger treatment difference, and a more definitive statement, than those using the unadjusted logrank statistic. This illustrates an important practical consideration, that only a small imbalance in an important prognostic factor can influence the conclusions drawn, even from reasonably large patient groups.

Other factors known to affect prognosis, such as clinical performance status, history of fits and extent of neurosurgery, were well balanced between the two treatment groups. Adjustment for these factors, in addition to age, did not alter the estimate of the treatment effect substantially from HR = 0.75.

6.13   ASSESSING PROPORTIONALITY OF HAZARDS

It is important that the proportional hazards assumption holds for valid interpretation of regression coefficients in a Cox model. A graphical check on the proportionality is provided by a complementary log plot over several values or

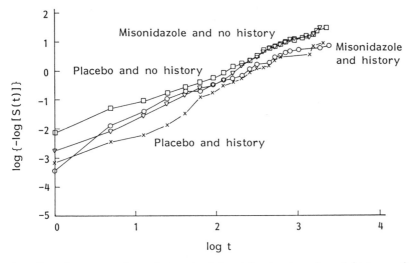

Figure 6.5 Complementary log plot against log t by treatment and history of fits for patients with brain tumours

grouped values of a variable, as has been indicated in Figures 6.1 and 6.2. The different values of the variables, presence or not of metastatic disease and limited or extensive disease in our examples, are reflected in separate, not necessarily 'parallel', lines in the complementary log plot. The technical reason for this is detailed below.

The survival function corresponding to the proportional hazards model of equation (6.12) can be expressed as

$$S(t;x) = S(t;x_0) \exp(\beta x) \tag{6.26}$$

where x and x_0 are values of the variables. In particular x_0 is the value of the variable in the baseline group. The x's are included here to emphasise their possible influence on survival. From equation (6.26) we have

$$\log\{-\log[S(t;x)]\} = \log\{-\log[S(t;x_0)]\} + \beta x. \tag{6.27}$$

As a consequence, a complementary log plot, which is a plot of the left-hand side of equation (6.27), against log t will give separate curves depending on the number of different values of the variable x. This is because the right-hand side of equation (6.27) has a part which varies with t, which is distinct from the part which varies with x. Any changes in the x term cause a step vertically up or down in the plot. The size of the step depends on the importance of the variable on prognosis.

If there are several variables, say, v in all, then βx is replaced in equation (6.27) by $\beta_1 x_1 + \beta_2 x_2 + \ldots + \beta_v x_v$. The corresponding plot will then have the possibility of many distinct curves.

Example

A check on the proportional hazards of the four treatment by history of fits graphs is provided by the complementary log plots of Figure 6.5. The parallel lines indicate approximately proportional hazards in the four patient groups. The differences in the lines suggest a relatively major difference in prognosis for those with and without a history of fits. In contrast the effect of treatment appears minimal.

6.14   TESTS AVAILABLE FOR ASSESSING MODELS

There are three principal tests available for assessing and comparing different models. These are the Wald test, the likelihood ratio test, and the score test. Although they are all equivalent if the number of events is large, for consistency and stability reasons in the associated methods of calculation the likelihood ratio test is preferred.

WALD TEST

As we have shown, when fitting a Cox model of a single variable x, which may be a binary variable or a continuous variable, we obtain an estimate, b, of the associated regression coefficient, β, together with the SE(b). The statistical significance of this variable, which is equivalent to a test of the null hypothesis, $\beta = 0$, is established by use of the $z = b/SE(b)$ test and of Table T1 of the Normal distribution. Equivalently, we can use the Wald test, where $W = z^2$, of equation (6.9), and Table T3 of the χ^2 distribution with df = 1.

This test can also be used to test if the addition of another variable, to a Cox model already containing v variables, improves the model. For example, the addition of the interaction term to the **F + G** model containing $v = 2$ variables of Table 6.7 was tested using this approach, but using z rather than W. In fact $W = z^2 = 0.17$ in this case. However, the test, in this situation, is only strictly valid if the estimated regression coefficients for the v variables are not unduly influenced by the presence of the additional variable. For example, b_F changes from -0.3924 to -0.3379, and b_G from 0.0144 to 0.0269 in Table 6.7 by the addition of the interaction term. We are then required to judge if these changes are substantial or not.

LIKELIHOOD RATIO TEST

The basis for a more general test than the Wald test, and one which can cope both with categorical variables of more than two levels and with adding several variables simultaneously to a Cox model, is the likelihood ratio (LR) test which we described in section 1.6.

A loose definition of the likelihood is that it is the probability of the observed data being 'explained' by a particular model. To illustrate this test, we first define the null model which, in the terminology of the Cox model, specifies that no variable influences survival. When the variable is treatment, this is equivalent to setting $\beta = 0$ in equation (6.5) to imply $\lambda_N(t) = \lambda_C(t) = \lambda_0(t)$, or that, irrespective of treatment, all patients have the same hazard $\lambda_0(t)$. The likelihood for this model is denoted as l_0 where l denotes likelihood and the zero represents the fact that all the regression coefficients are set as zero.

In contrast, the likelihood of the model which contains v different regression coefficients is written as l_v and the regression coefficients are estimated by the method of maximum likelihood. The larger l_v is relative to l_0, the better the model explains, or fits, the observed data.

The fit of each model can be tested using the likelihood ratio (LR) or

$$LR = -2 \log(l_0/l_v)$$
$$= -2(L_0 - L_v) \qquad (6.28)$$

where $L_v = \log l_v$ and $L_0 = \log l_0$. This is in the same form as equation (1.14) with suffix v replacing suffix a. We can think of the Cox model containing v variables as the alternative hypothesis and that containing no variables as the null hypothesis.

Under the hypothesis of no difference in the two models, i.e. where including the variables in the Cox model does not help to explain the survival data any more satisfactorily than the null model with no variables, the LR of equation (6.28) has a χ^2 distribution with degrees of freedom df = v.

To assess the relative fit of two models, one with (v + k) regression coefficients and the other with fewer, say, v regression coefficients, we can use the statistic

$$LR = 2(L_{v+k} - L_v). \qquad (6.29)$$

This statistic also has a χ^2 distribution, but with df = (v + k) − v = k. The null hypothesis here is that there is no improvement in the fit of the model, by including the extra k coefficients.

Example

We noted in Table 6.7 that $\chi^2 = 11.69$ for the main effects model $F + G$. This is, in fact, better described as LR = 11.69 which, under the null hypothesis or model (1), has a χ^2 distribution with v = 2 degrees of freedom. Use of Table T3 with df = 2 suggests a corresponding p-value between 0.01 and 0.001, since 11.69 is between the tabular values of 9.21 and 13.82. More detailed tables of the χ^2 distribution give a p-value ≈ 0.005. From this we conclude that the main effects model is an improvement over the null model.

SCORE TEST

The score test, S, is, in the case of a single binary variable, the same as the Mantel–Haenszel version of the logrank test of equation (4.11). In situations with continuous variables and/or more than one variable in a model, it is a generalisation of this test.

The form of the S test is complex. In brief, however, the numerator in the calculation of S is the square of the first derivative of the log likelihood, L. We gave an example of L in equation (1.13) and referred to its derivative in section 1.7 and in equation (3.18). This numerator is then evaluated, with the parameters of interest in our model all set to zero.

The denominator of S is the second derivative of L, which is also evaluated with the parameters of interest set to zero. This latter term is called the information and is essentially an estimate of the variance. The resulting ratio of the numerator and denominator is S, which has a χ^2 distribution, with an appropriate number of degrees of freedom.

Example

For the 417 patients with brain cancer, the equivalent score statistic for the two-factor model $F + G$ of Table 6.7 is $S = 11.69$. Note that, in this situation, this is exactly equivalent to the LR statistic and it too has a χ^2 distribution with $df = 2$. Thus, in this case, the same p-value is also obtained for the fit of the model.

We return to the problem of testing the statistical significance of individual regression coefficients in a Cox model in chapter 7.

Selecting Variables within a Cox Model

Summary

For use in practice, a Cox proportional hazards model needs to contain as few variables as possible, yet must still describe the data as adequately as possible. Such a model is termed parsimonious. Thus, an important problem is how variables in a Cox model are selected for inclusion or exclusion, in situations in which there are several, perhaps many, possible variables to choose from. We describe the step-up, step-down and all combinations methods of selecting the final variables to include in the model. Although our concern here is with the Cox model, the problems associated with selecting variables are similar for other multiple regression techniques.

7.1 INTRODUCTION

Suppose the data of Table 6.1 did not arise from a randomised clinical trial, but merely recorded some characteristics of patients with brain cancer. These patients are then followed from a well-defined time point, say initial diagnosis, until death. In this situation, the object of the study may be to identify, by means of a Cox model, which if any of these recorded characteristics are important in predicting the subsequent prognosis of patients. Once determined, knowledge of these characteristics and hence the subsequent prognosis may help in the counselling of future patients with brain cancer and may also influence the choice of therapy for them. For example, advice and/or treatment may differ for those with good or bad prognosis. We assume that if a variable has little or no prognostic consequence, we would not want it in our model.

To illustrate the procedure, we use the 205 patients of the standard (control) group of brain cancer patients who received radiotherapy alone for their disease (section 4.8). Again, for illustration purposes, we assume that there are only three potential prognostic variables: history of fits (F), tumour grade (G) and age (A), recorded at diagnosis. We ignore the possibility of any interaction terms between any of the variables. For discussion purposes, we shall regard all three variables as binary: history of fits (No, Yes), grade (3 and 3/4, 4), age (less than 50, 50+). For the three variables of interest, the eight possible proportional hazards models are summarised in Table 7.1.

We use a shorthand description of these eight models. One standard way is to refer to the null model as model (1), and the remaining models using the full capital letter of the variable names involved; here F, G and A, as we have done previously in section 5.5 and chapter 6. The letters on their own depict the one-variable model which consists of that variable alone. Thus, model F includes history of fits, but no other variables. In an obvious notation, model F + G includes history of fits and grade, while model A + F includes age and history of fits. The model F + G + A includes all three variables. The order we place F, G or A in any model using this notation is not important. The β's within each model of Table 7.1 are the regression coefficients and the x's the values of the associated, potentially prognostic, variables.

To illustrate the various methods for selecting variables for inclusion in a Cox model, these eight models have each been fitted to the data from the 205 control patients with brain cancer, 198 of whom had died at the time of analysis. The remaining seven still alive provide censored observations in this example. The details of the fitted models are given in Table 7.2.

We now have to choose which of these models best describes our data. For example, should we choose model F rather than model F + G + A? We might be

Table 7.1 Possible Cox models for three potentially prognostic variables (history of fits, grade and age) for patients with a brain cancer

Model	Notation	Equation for $h = \lambda(t)/\lambda_0(t)$
Null	(1)	1
One-variable		
History of Fits	F	$\exp(\beta_F x_F)$
Grade	G	$\exp(\beta_G x_G)$
Age	A	$\exp(\beta_A x_A)$
Two-variable		
History of Fits and Grade	F + G	$\exp(\beta_F x_F + \beta_G x_G)$
Grade and Age	G + A	$\exp(\beta_G x_G + \beta_A x_A)$
Age and History of Fits	A + F	$\exp(\beta_A x_A + \beta_F x_F)$
Three-variable		
History of Fits, Grade and Age	F + G + A	$\exp(\beta_F x_F + \beta_G x_G + \beta_A x_A)$

Table 7.2 Cox models, using the three binary factors: history of fits, grade and age fitted to survival data from patients with brain cancer receiving radiotherapy alone for their disease (From Medical Research Council Working Party on Misonidazole in Gliomas, 1983. Reproduced by permission of The British Institute of Radiology.)

Variables		No variables	One variable			Two variables			Three variables
		(1)	F	G	A	F+G	G+A	A+F	F+G+A
History of Fits									
(No, Yes)	b	—	-0.4840	—	—	-0.4875	—	-0.4647	-0.4684
	SE(b)	—	0.1715	—	—	0.1718	—	0.1720	0.1730
	HR	—	0.6163	—	—	0.6142	—	0.6284	0.6260
	W	—	7.97	—	—	8.05	—	7.30	7.33
	P	—	0.0048	—	—	0.0046	—	0.0069	0.0068
Grade									
(3 and 3/4, 4)	b	—	—	0.0321	—	0.0552	-0.0142	—	0.0300
	SE(b)	—	—	0.1436	—	0.1439	0.1441	—	0.1446
	HR	—	—	1.0327	—	1.0568	0.9859	—	1.0304
	W	—	—	0.05	—	0.15	0.01	—	0.04
	P	—	—	0.8228	—	0.7011	0.9212	—	0.8357
Age (years)									
(<50, ≥50)	b	—	—	—	0.6633	—	0.6645	0.6528	0.6513
	SE(b)	—	—	—	0.1569	—	0.1574	0.1575	0.1577
	HR	—	—	—	1.9411	—	1.9434	1.9209	1.9181
	W	—	—	—	17.88	—	17.83	17.17	17.07
	P	—	—	—	<0.0001	—	<0.0001	<0.0001	<0.0001
	$-2 \log l$	1760.76	1752.14	1760.71	1741.89	1751.99	1741.88	1734.02	1733.98
	LR		8.62	0.05	18.87	8.77	18.88	26.74	26.78
	p-value		0.0033	0.8231	<0.0001	0.012	<0.0001	<0.0001	<0.0001

tempted to do so, since **F** has fewer terms and is, therefore, simpler than **F** + **G** + **A**. However, we may then be concerned that we have excluded possibly useful information from factors **G** and **A**, which may be of importance in determining prognosis. We now describe several approaches to help us make the final choice.

7.2 STEP-UP SELECTION

SIMPLE APPROACH

A step-up variable selection procedure adds one variable at a time to the current model.

Step I

The first step is to check if any of the models **F**, **G** or **A** is an improvement over the null model. That is, are any of these single-variable models an improvement over model (1)? Thus, we ask: are any of these models better than a model which contains no variables? We look to see which, if any, of the one-variable models has a statistically significant regression coefficient. This is done by use of either the Wald (W) or likelihood ratio (LR) tests, described in section 6.14.

The 'One variable' panel of Table 7.2 gives the W and LR statistics for the three one-variable models. We begin by focusing on the W test. The associated p-values for the W statistic of the models **F**, **G** and **A** are 0.0048, 0.8228 and < 0.0001, respectively. The p-values quoted were obtained by use of Table T1 of the Normal distribution rather than Table T3 of the χ^2 distribution. This is because $z = \sqrt{W}$, and W has df = 1.

One simple way of selecting a single-variable model is to consider whether a variable has an associated p-value ≤ 0.05. On this basis, we would exclude model **G** as it does not reach this conventional statistical significance, since the p-value = 0.8228, which is clearly > 0.05. Had, in addition, neither **F** nor **A** an associated p-value ≤ 0.05, then we would have retained our null model (1) as the final model. In such a situation, we would conclude that none of the three variables under consideration appear to help in predicting survival duration in these patients; i.e., they do not appear to be prognostic for the disease.

However, in our example, both models **F** and **A** have an associated p-value < 0.05. This suggests that one of these models might be used and, therefore, the null model containing no prognostic variables is clearly not appropriate. We now have to decide between models **F** and **A**. One method is to take, as the first prognostic variable of our model, the variable which has the smallest associated p-value. This corresponds to model **A** with a p-value < 0.0001. Thus, our Step I model for describing these data includes age alone and is

$$\textbf{A: } h = \exp(0.6633 x_A). \tag{7.1}$$

In this model, $x_A = 0$ corresponds to the younger patients of less than 50 years and $x_A = 1$ to those who are ≥ 50. The corresponding HR for age, from Table 7.2, is 1.94, which indicates almost twice the death rate amongst the older women. The corresponding HRs for a history of fits and tumour grade are 0.62 and 1.03, respectively. These indicate a lower risk for patients with a history of fits and a higher risk for those with Grade 4 tumours. However, both of these hazard ratios are closer to HR = 1, than the HR for age.

In this example, the binary variable age at diagnosis appears very important to the duration of these patients' subsequent survival. This is illustrated in the Kaplan–Meier plots of Figure 7.1 for the two age groups, indicating a median survival of approximately 11 months for the younger patients and only 6 months for the older.

Step II

The next question to ask is: do any of the remaining variables if added to the model, already including age, help to explain the variation between patients further? If not, then equation (7.1) becomes the final model, otherwise we seek to add a further variable to this model.

In this case, there are two possible models, **G + A** and **A + F**, that we need to consider. The model **F + G** is not considered here as it does not contain age. This is because Step I has suggested that age is an important variable and, therefore, should be included in any final model.

The 'Two variables' panel of Table 7.2 gives W = 7.30 for the estimated regression coefficient for history of fits in model **A + F** and a corresponding p-value = 0.0069. In contrast, W = 0.01 for the estimated regression coefficient for tumour grade in model **G + A**, with a p-value = 0.92. This therefore suggests that at Step II we add

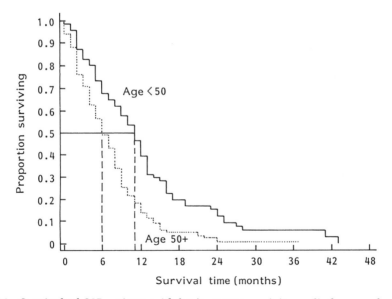

Figure 7.1 Survival of 205 patients with brain cancer receiving radiotherapy alone by age group (From Medical Research Council Working Party on Misonidazole in Gliomas, 1983. Reproduced by permission of The British Institute of Radiology.)

history of fits to the Step I model containing age alone. The one-variable model is now extended and is replaced by

$$\textbf{A} + \textbf{F}: h = \exp(0.6528x_A - 0.4647x_F). \tag{7.2}$$

Here $x_F = 0$ for those who have no history of fits and $x_F = 1$ for those with a history. The survival of patients from the four age by history of fits groups is illustrated in Figure 7.2, which suggests some differences in survival between the four patient groups. In particular, patients who are aged less than 50, with a history of fits, have the best prognosis and a median survival time of approximately 1 year. We conclude, at this second step, that the additional knowledge concerning a patient's history of fits gives further prognostic information over that provided by age alone.

We note that the estimated regression coefficient for age, $b_A = 0.6528$, in equation (7.2) of model $\textbf{A} + \textbf{F}$, has altered slightly in numerical value from $b_A = 0.6633$, derived in Step I to obtain model $\textbf{A}$ of equation (7.1).

Step III

The next step in our procedure is to decide if we need to advance to the final model $\textbf{F} + \textbf{G} + \textbf{A}$, which includes all the potential prognostic variables. For that model, included in the last column of Table 7.2, the coefficients for age and history of fits are significant using the W test, but that for grade is not. These suggest that we do not include grade in the model and have no need to go beyond the two-variable model $\textbf{A} + \textbf{F}$ to describe the data.

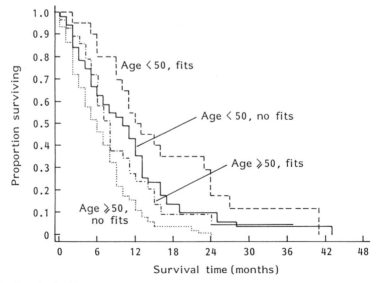

Figure 7.2 Survival of brain cancer patients receiving radiotherapy alone by the four age by history of fits groups (From Medical Research Council Working Party on Misonidazole in Gliomas, 1983. Reproduced by permission of The British Institute of Radiology.)

We conclude from this modelling process that both age and history of fits together may be useful in helping to predict prognosis, whereas adding information on tumour grade to these is unlikely to be useful.

It should be noticed that the values of the regression coefficients for age and history of fits, in model $F + G + A$, differ from the corresponding values in equation (7.2), albeit only marginally.

BETTER APPROACH

We have used the simple approach merely as an illustration of the principles of a step-up procedure. It is not, however, the best procedure to adopt. The main problem is that it does not include a measure of how good the respective models are in explaining the variation. A good model will be one which explains the variation within the data leaving as little unexplained variation as possible. We therefore need to assess whether a particular model reduces the unexplained variation by a significant amount. To do this we need to assess whether it increases the likelihood, l, by a significant amount, or equivalently reduces $-2 \log l$ by a significant amount, as we have indicated in section 6.14.

For example, to compare the fit of model F of Table 7.2 with that of the null model (1), we calculate, using equations similar to (6.28) and (6.29), the LR as

$$
\begin{aligned}
LR_{F,(1)} &= (-2 \log l_{(1)}) - (-2 \log l_F) \\
&= -2(L_{(1)} - L_F) \\
&= 2(L_F - L_{(1)}).
\end{aligned} \tag{7.3}
$$

We note a change in the notation from that adopted earlier in equations (6.28) and (6.29), in that the subscripts to L used here are the models under consideration rather than their degrees of freedom. In this case, we use bold case for the subscript to distinguish from the degrees of freedom used earlier, where we use a standard font for the subscript. These notations are used interchangeably, depending on the context. We also note that we have attached a description of the models being compared as a subscript to the LR of the left-hand side of equation (7.3). This is done for ease of presentation.

The number of degrees of freedom for each model is the number of observed events, O, minus the number of regression coefficients included in the model. Thus, for the model F, there are $v = 1$ regression coefficients fitted, the observed number of deaths, $O = 205 - 7 = 198$, and hence $df = O - v = 198 - 1 = 197$. In a similar way, the degrees of freedom for the null model, (1), are $198 - 0 = 198$. This is because no regression coefficients are estimated. The degrees of freedom for $LR_{F,(1)}$ are, therefore, the difference between these two sets, i.e. $df = 198 - 197 = 1$.

This is, in fact, the difference in the number of parameters in model F, which is 1, and the number of parameters in model (1), which is 0. Thus, under the null hypothesis that fitting the model F does not explain any more of the variation in the data than the null model, $LR_{F,(1)}$ has a χ^2 distribution with $df = 1$.

The rule for calculating the degrees of freedom for the comparison of two models, by subtracting the number of parameters fitted in the two models, is a general one, provided the models are nested. Two models are nested if the model with the larger number of variables includes, amongst these variables, all the variables of the smaller model. Thus, for example, model **A** is nested in model **F + G + A**, but it is not nested in model **F + G**.

If we wish to compare the model **F + G** with the model **F**, then we would calculate the corresponding LR statistic, which is

$$LR_{F+G,F} = LR_{F+G,(1)} - LR_{F,(1)}. \tag{7.4}$$

We can generalise equation (7.4) and state that in order to obtain the LR statistic for comparing two models, we subtract the two LR statistics obtained by comparing each of the models in turn with the null model. Under the null hypothesis, that the larger model does not reduce the variation in the data, as compared to the nested model containing fewer terms, the LR statistic again follows a χ^2 distribution. The degrees of freedom are equal to the difference in the number of parameters contained in the two models, as indicated earlier.

Returning to the data for the 205 patients with brain tumours, the LR statistics comparing each model with the null model are included in Table 7.2 and are also shown in the second column of Table 7.3.

We also calculate the difference between the LR statistics for the two-variable models, using the equivalent of equation (7.4). In this way we obtain the LR statistic for each of the three comparisons of the two-variable and corresponding nested one-variable models. Thus, comparing model **F + G** with individual models **F** and **G** in turn gives $LR_{F+G,F} = 8.77 - 8.62 = 0.15$ and $LR_{F+G,G} = 8.77 - 0.05 = 8.72$. In a similar way, model **F + G + A** is compared to each of the three two-variable models. In this case, all three models are nested within model **F + G + A**. All nine LR statistics are given in the main body of Table 7.3.

Finally, we note that the LRs for the models **F**, **G** and **A** are close, but not always

Table 7.3 Likelihood ratio (LR) statistics and degrees of freedom (df) for all possible models, including history of fits, tumour grade and age for patients with brain cancer (From Medical Research Council Working Party for Misonidazole in Gliomas, 1983. Reproduced by permission of The British Institute of Radiology.)

| | | | LR statistics | | | |
| | | | Two variables | | | Three variables |
Model	LR with the null model	df	F + G	G + A	A + F	F + G + A
(1)	–	198	–	–	–	–
F	8.62	197	0.15	–	18.12	–
G	0.05	197	8.72	18.83	–	–
A	18.87	197	–	0.01	7.87	–
F + G	8.77	196	–	–	–	18.01
G + A	18.88	196	–	–	–	7.90
A + F	26.74	196	–	–	–	0.04
F + G + A	26.78	195	–	–	–	–

exactly equal, to the comparable W statistic of Table 7.2. This will usually be the case. Once all the relevant LRs are calculated, the variable selection procedure is then applied as follows.

Step I

From Table 7.3, we see that fitting model **A** gives a $LR_{A,(1)} = 18.87$ against the null model (1) with no variables in it. This has a χ^2 distribution with df = 1 and, thus, from Table T3 we have a p-value <0.0005. This is considerably less than 0.05, the conventional level for statistical significance, and suggests that an improvement over the null model would be achieved by including age. If we consider the other models with just one variable, then for model **F** we have $LR_{F,(1)} = 8.62$, df = 1, which has, from Table T3, a p-value <0.01. Similarly, model **G** gives $LR_{G,(1)} = 0.05$, again with df = 1 and a p-value >0.2, which in this case is larger than 0.05. By analogy with the situation of the W test, exact values for these p-values can be obtained by referring $\sqrt{LR}$ to Table T1, since df = 1. This gives for models **F** and **G** exact p-values of 0.0044 and 0.8228, respectively. These are both larger than that for model **A** and thus our best model at Step I is model **A**.

Step II

For the second step, we calculate the LRs corresponding to the differences between models **A** and **A** + **F** and between models **A** and **G** + **A**. These are indicated in Table 7.3 and give $LR_{A+F,A} = 26.74 - 18.87 = 7.87$ and $LR_{A+G,A} = 18.88 - 18.87 = 0.01$, which each have df = 1. The corresponding p-values are 0.0050 and 0.92, respectively. These suggest that, whereas adding **F** to the Step I model of **A** alone 'improves the fit' and therefore gives a better model, adding **G** does not improve the model. Our Step II model is therefore **A** + **F**.

Step III

The final step is to calculate the LR between model **F** + **G** + **A** and model **A** + **F**. This is given in Table 7.3 by $LR_{F+G+A,A+F} = 26.78 - 26.74 = 0.04$, with corresponding p-value = 0.84. This comparison implies that grade does not reduce the unexplained variation significantly and so does not add any further information. The 'best' and final model for our data is thus **A** + **F**.

This procedure results in the same final model that we had derived previously using the simple approach. However, this will not always be the case.

7.3   STEP-DOWN SELECTION

Step I

In contrast to the step-up procedures, which start with the null model (1), the step-down procedure starts with the full model **F** + **G** + **A** fitted to the data. Thus, from the final column of Table 7.2, we begin with

$$\mathbf{F} + \mathbf{G} + \mathbf{A}: h = \exp(-0.4684x_F + 0.0300x_G + 0.6513x_A). \tag{7.5}$$

We now check if this model is an improvement over the null model, by considering the LR statistic $LR_{F+G+A,(1)} = 26.78$ of Tables 7.2 and 7.3.

Under the null hypothesis, that this model containing all three variables is no improvement over the null model containing no variables, the LR statistic has a χ^2 distribution with df $= 3$, which is equal to the number of parameters in model $F + G + A$. Reference to Table T3 with $LR_{F+G+A,(1)} = 26.78$, df $= 3$, gives a p-value <0.0005. Thus, there is evidence that this model is an improvement over the null model. Our Step I model is therefore $F + G + A$.

If the p-value had not been statistically significant, then we would have adopted the model containing no variables, i.e. model (1). The selection procedure would have then been terminated at Step I.

Step II

The next step checks if any one of the variables contained in the full model can be removed from the model without serious loss of fit. Thus, we calculate the corresponding LR statistics by comparing the three-variable model $F + G + A$ with each of the two-variable models $F + G$, $A + F$ and $G + A$ in turn. The smallest of these three LR statistics, provided it is not statistically significant at a predefined significance level, would indicate that the corresponding variable should be dropped from the full model. The argument here is that if the likelihood is not changed much by omitting a particular variable, then we would prefer to describe the data using a model containing as few variables as possible.

In our example, the respective LRs are $LR_{F+G+A,F+G} = 26.78 - 8.77 = 18.01$, $LR_{F+G+A,A+F} = 26.78 - 26.74 = 0.04$ and $LR_{F+G+A,G+A} = 26.78 - 18.88 = 7.90$. These are included in the final column of Table 7.3. The smallest of these is $LR_{F+G+A,A+F} = 0.04$, with df $= 3 - 2 = 1$. This gives a p-value of 0.84, which is much larger than the conventional level of significance of 0.05. Thus, inclusion of G in the model is not regarded as adding much information. As a consequence, we remove G from the Step I model to give model $A + F$ as our Step II model.

Had all three LR statistics considered here been statistically significant, we would have retained the full model $F + G + A$ and gone no further in the selection process.

Step III

The next step is to compare model $A + F$ with the nested single variable models A and F separately to obtain $LR_{A+F,F} = 26.74 - 8.62 = 18.12$ and $LR_{A+F,A} = 26.74 - 18.87 = 7.87$, both of which have df $= 1$. The corresponding p-values obtained by use of Table T3 are <0.0005 and <0.01. Thus, these p-values are considerably less than 0.05 for both comparisons. This indicates that if we omit either of these variables from the Step II model we may seriously affect the fit of the model. Our final model, therefore, remains as

$$A + F: h = \exp(-0.4647x_F + 0.6528x_A). \tag{7.6}$$

This is the same final model as that resulting from both the procedures described previously.

Table 7.4 Likelihood ratio (LR) statistics and degrees of freedom (df) of all possible models compared to the null model for the survival data from patients receiving radiotherapy treatment for their brain cancer (From Medical Research Council Working Party on Misonidazole in Gliomas, 1983. Reproduced by permission of The British Institute of Radiology.)

Model	Model df	LR	LR df	p-value
F	197	8.62	1	0.0033
G	197	0.05	1	0.8231
A	197	18.87	1	0.000014
F + G	196	8.77	2	0.01246
G + A	196	18.88	2	0.000079
A + F	196	26.74	2	0.0000016
F + G + A	195	26.78	3	0.0000066

7.4 ALL POSSIBLE COMBINATIONS

A third option for selecting models is to compare the null model (1) with every other possible model and to calculate the corresponding LR statistics against this null model. These LRs were given in the second column of Table 7.3, but are reproduced in Table 7.4 for convenience, together with their associated degrees of freedom and exact p-values. As before, the values of the LR statistics are compared with a χ^2 distribution, using the appropriate degrees of freedom. The exact p-values corresponding to df = 2 and df = 3 were obtained as part of the output of a statistical package used for fitting the Cox models and not from Table T3.

Quite simply, we choose the best model from the seven models of Table 7.4 as that with the smallest associated p-value. This gives the same model as before, i.e. A + F with p-value = 0.0000016. If none of the p-values in Table 7.4 had been <0.05, then this all combinations method would give model (1) for our data set.

7.5 CHOICE OF SELECTION METHOD

As already indicated, the method we refer to as 'simple' is not a recommended procedure since it does not include a criterion for assessing the reduction in variation arising from a comparison between alternative models. Thus, we are left with the step-up (better approach), step-down and all combination options. In general, the 'all combination' method would be preferable in that every model is examined and, therefore, one is not going to miss the 'best' model merely because it has not been looked at.

We should note, however, that although we have used real data in our example, we have chosen the three particular variables and expressed these in binary form for illustrative purposes only. In practice, there were more than 15 variables recorded at diagnosis from these patients, all of which were potential candidates for prognostic consideration. These give a possibility of $2^{15} = 32\,768$ different models to choose from if all variables are treated as binary. In this case, the 'all combinations' selection method is not practicable as it would require too much computing time to implement. The step-down procedure can also be ruled out, as we would first fit a model for the 15 variables, i.e. the model $F + G + A + B + C + \ldots + N$, where the letters **B** through to **N**, omitting **F** for history of fits and **G** for tumour grade, are labels for the other 12 variables. Even with a total of 402 deaths in the combined data set, there are clearly too few events for such an extensive model to be fitted. In such a situation, we are left with the 'step-up' procedure as the only practicable possibility.

A compromise, in some situations where there are many possible models, is first to fit all the possible one-variable models, i.e. fit the individual models **F, G, A, B, ..., N**, respectively. We then only consider, as possible candidates for the selection procedure, those variables which have significant regression coefficients at that stage. If this preliminary screening removes many of the variables from the selection process, then one can go to the 'all combinations' method, which is now confined to this reduced subset of variables.

7.6   WHICH SIGNIFICANCE LEVEL?

As for many statistical procedures, the choice of the level to decide between 'significant' and 'non-significant' is a subjective matter. Again, as for many procedures, the 0.05 level is often used. However, another common level used in selecting variables for inclusion in a Cox model is 0.1. The reason for this is, that with such a level, we are less likely to reject a possibly important variable. When building a model, it may be better to err on the side of caution, i.e. to include a variable rather than exclude it. This is especially the case during the early stages, for example, in the variable by variable screening procedure, mentioned above. This caution may also be important if, as can happen, the 'significance' of an individual variable is enhanced when it is combined with other variables. In any case, little may be lost if a less stringent level is used at the early stages, since if the variable is in truth of little importance, it will drop out of the model at a later stage.

7.7   CATEGORICAL AND CONTINUOUS VARIABLES

As we have indicated for categorical variables of g levels, it is often necessary to create $g - 1$ dummy variables for utilisation in a Cox model. Some caution must also be taken if one is incorporating a categorical variable of three (or more) levels into an automatic selection procedure. Thus, in the illustrative example of this chapter, if we were to include a factor **G** with the three brain tumour grade categories recorded as 3, 3/4 and 4, then we need to specify two dummy variables in the associated model. We do this in the way we described in equation (6.22) of section 6.9. In this situation, we must constrain the selection procedure always to consider the pair of dummy variables together. If grade is not predictive of prognosis, then both dummy variables would be excluded from the model. If grade is predictive, then both dummy variables are retained in the model. In some statistical packages, all that is necessary to ensure this is to declare that the variable is categorical with g groups. The program then creates the dummy variables automatically and, most importantly, will either include or not include, as appropriate, all dummy variables for that categorical variable in any model.

Although we have treated age as a binary categorical variable in this chapter, this is not desirable, in general, as information is lost. In addition, if a reduction of a continuous variable to a binary variable is made, then this implies a discrete jump from 1 to $\exp(\beta)$ in the hazard at the breakpoint, for example at a patient's 50th birthday. This step-up, or step-down, of the hazard at the cut point is likely to be unrealistic in practice, as one might expect a smooth transition of the hazard with changing values rather than an abrupt change.

If a categorisation is thought desirable, and this will depend on the medical context, then it is best if at least three categories are created.

Example from the literature

The women included in the investigation by the World Health Organization Task Force on Long-acting Systems Agents for Fertility Regulation (1990) are divided into four weight groups as in Table 5.5. Such an ordered categorisation allows examination of trend. The trend may be approximately linear, as in the association between the number of pregnancies and body weight in those women using a vaginal ring for contraceptive purposes. On the other hand, the trend may be non-linear, in circumstances where, for example, the intermediate categories have higher (or lower) risk than the categories above and below.

In general, we would prefer to model a variable such as age as a continuous variable if possible, as in equation (6.15). However, such a model also has its problems, as it implies that the effect of age is linear over the whole range of possible values, from the youngest patient with a brain tumour to the oldest. This may not always be the case. One method of checking for linearity is to divide age, at the preliminary stage of analysis, into $g \geq 3$ categories and to fit a dummy variable model. If a plot of the resulting $(g-1)$ regression coefficients against the corresponding age category—a similar plot to that of Figure 6.4—is approximately linear, then we may assume that the influence of age may also be regarded as linear for our continuous model.

On the other hand, if such a graph does indicate some non-linearity, but the change in hazard is smooth from category to category, then one model that could be used to describe such a pattern is

$$\mathbf{A*A}: \ h_{A \cdot A} = \exp(\beta_A A + \beta_{A.A} A^2) \tag{7.7}$$

The model is denoted here by $\mathbf{A*A}$ as an abbreviation for $\mathbf{A + A.A}$. We noted earlier that the model of equation (6.24) which is $\mathbf{I + R + I.R}$ can be written as $\mathbf{I*R}$.

In mathematical terms, equation (7.7) is the equation of a parabola, or more usually termed a quadratic, since it contains a squared (in age) term. The model enables us to try to describe data with a smooth 'bend' in one direction.

Formally, we check the extra fit provided by this model over the linear model of equation (6.15), by testing the null hypothesis, $\beta_{A.A} = 0$. The procedure is the same as that for comparing any two nested models, which we described earlier. Thus, we calculate $LR_{A*A.A}$ and this has a χ^2 distribution with $df = 1$. The latter is because equation (7.7) contains two parameters β_A and $\beta_{A.A}$, while equation (6.15) has only one parameter, β_A. Hence, $df = 2 - 1 = 1$.

There is a distinction, however, between this situation and that when we are deciding, for example, between models $A + F$ and models A or F individually. In the latter case, model A or model F is nested within the full model and both are candidates to replace $A + F$. In contrast, in the situation when testing for linearity, there is only one alternative to $A*A$ and that is model A, which is nested within it. It is useful to check if this is the selection procedure adopted by the computer package being used for the analysis. Some packages define a new variable, say $U = A^2$, then fit the model $A + U$, without any regard to the basic structure of equation (7.7). In this formulation model U is regarded as one of the possibilities for the final model. This is an inappropriate procedure.

We note that the quadratic equation (7.7) is also termed a polynomial of order 2. It can be extended to a polynominal of any power of age by, for example

$$h_v = \exp(\beta_1 A + \beta_2 A^2 + \dots + \beta_{v-1} A^{v-1} + \beta_v A^v). \tag{7.8}$$

Such an equation has v regression coefficients, $\beta_1, \beta_2, \dots, \beta_v$, and is termed a polynomial in age of order v. This model can be fitted to an appropriate data set and nested models of order less than v compared, using the LR test that we have described.

Example from the literature

Umen and Le (1986) described a study investigating survival of patients with end-stage renal disease. They derive models including age, presence or absence of arteriosclerotic heart disease (ASHD), cerebrovascular accident (CVA), cancer (CA) and chronic obstructive pulmonary disease (COPD) for non-diabetic patients in their study, but find a model including age alone as appropriate for diabetic patients.

Their models, derived by considering a larger group of models containing up to 16 potentially prognostic variables, are summarised in Table 7.5. To determine which variables to include, they screened each variable individually and in combination with others, and then eliminated those variables that failed to generate a p-value ≤ 0.1. Using those variables remaining after this initial screen, they used a step-wise forward selection process to achieve the final models.

In both models, age is regarded as a three-group categorical variable requiring two dummy variables in the modelling process. In the patients who do not have diabetes, a comparison of those patients aged 1–45 years with the oldest patients of 61 or more years, used as the reference group, gives $HR = \exp(-1.576) = 0.21$. This indicates a much reduced risk of death for the younger group of patients. In those patients with diabetes, the same comparison between the youngest and oldest age groups gives $HR = \exp(-0.676) = 0.51$. This also provides evidence of a reduced

Table 7.5 Cox regression models for survival in end-stage renal disease for patients with and without diabetes (From Umen and Le, 1986 with permission)

	Non-diabetic patients			Diabetic patients		
	Regression coefficient	SE	HR	Regression coefficient	SE	HR
Age (1–45)	−1.576	0.402	0.21	−0.676	0.307	0.51
(46–60)	−0.644	0.238	0.53	−0.569	0.313	0.57
ASHD	0.424	0.178	1.53	–	–	–
CVA	0.741	0.254	2.10	–	–	–
CA	0.441	0.212	1.55	–	–	–
COPD	0.452	0.199	1.57	–	–	–

risk, but is not of the magnitude of that observed in those without diabetes. This suggests that there may be an interaction between the presence or absence of diabetes and age.

The HRs associated with ASHD, CVA, CA and COPD are all greater than unity. The presence of any of these indicates an increased risk of death for non-diabetic patients with end-stage renal cancer. These same variables were not found to influence survival amongst the diabetic patients.

7.8   INTERACTION TERMS

Suppose we were investigating the possible interaction between patient age (**A**) and history of fits (**F**) on survival of patients with brain cancer. In this investigation, we conjecture that the survival advantage of those with a history of fits, as opposed to those who do not have a history, may not be of the same magnitude in the two-patient age groups (<50 and ≥50 years). Thus, the prognostic influence of history of fits may be dependent on the age of the patient at diagnosis. We may wish to test this conjecture by means of a Cox model.

We will assume here that both **A** and **F** are important for our model. We could test for the presence of an interaction by fitting model **A∗F**, i.e. model **A + F + A.F**, to the data and comparing it with model **A + F**. It is then necessary to calculate $LR_{A*F,A+F}$, which will have a χ^2 distribution with df = 1.

In formal terms we have, by analogy with equation (6.24), the interaction model as

$$\textbf{A∗F: } h = \exp(\beta_A x_A + \beta_F x_F + \beta_{AF} x_A x_F). \tag{7.9}$$

in this situation, a test for the presence of an interaction is equivalent to testing the null hypothesis that the regression coefficient $\beta_{AF} = 0$.

Again, it is useful to check that if this model is fitted using a selection procedure, then the method adopted by the computer package does not have the potential to exclude either β_A, β_F or both, yet still retain the coefficient β_{AF} in the final model.

Thus, by analogy with the quadratic term for age, care should be taken to distinguish model $A*F$ from model $A + F + U$, where $U = A.F$ and $x_U = x_A x_F$. In this latter case, the automatic selection procedure may choose between $A + F$, $A + U$ and $F + U$ as alternatives to what appears to be a three-factor model, $A + F + U$; whereas the only sensible alternative to model $A*F$ of equation (7.9) is the model $A + F$. Here, model $A + F$ is nested within model $A*F$, but models $A + U$ and $F + U$ are not.

Example from the literature

In the study described by Umen and Le (1986), we suggested that there was evidence for an interaction between age and presence or absence of diabetes. This led the authors to develop two separate models: one for those patients without diabetes and the other for those with diabetes. They did this in preference to developing just a single model including a diagnosis by age interaction term. Their modelling approach was further complicated by the other four variables of Table 7.5 having a major influence on survival in non-diabetic patients, but having little influence on those with diabetes, as we indicated previously.

7.9   INFLUENCE OF OTHER VARIABLES ON REGRESSION COEFFICIENTS

We have indicated that the estimates of the regression coefficients can vary, depending on the presence or absence of other variables included in the model. Thus, the coefficient for age in Table 7.2 is 0.6633 in model A, 0.6528 in model $A + F$, 0.6645 in model $G + A$ and finally 0.6513 in model $F + G + A$. Although the changes are not large in this example, they can be substantial in some situations.

The changes are due to the presence of some statistical association between age and tumour grade, and age and history of fits. For example, older patients may have a tendency to have worse grades, merely since they are older. Also, chance alone can provide some association between variables. This will then lead to small differences in the values of the respective regression coefficients in models in which they are included together compared to those in which they are considered separately.

Any association implies that the two variables do not act independently, at least within the data set under consideration. If the variables were truly independent, their presence or absence in the model would not affect the others. If the association is large, then substantial changes will occur in the regression coefficients, depending on whether only one or both variables are in the model.

In fact, such association can lead to variables, already chosen for the model, being dropped at a later stage in the modelling process. To avoid this difficulty, it is often recommended that the data are first screened for association, perhaps by a scatter plot of one against the other, before modelling begins. If two variables are strongly associated with each other, then only one should be included in the modelling process. The single variable to be included should be chosen by considerations outside the modelling process. For example, there may be two alternative measures of a blood characteristic which are 'by definition' strongly associated. If one is easier to obtain than the other, then it may be that the easier one's influence is then the one to be tested in the Cox model. A separate study may be needed to choose which is the 'best' measure, but this should not be decided using a modelling process which includes other variables.

7.10 REPORTING SELECTION PROCEDURES

The modelling selection procedure used should be carefully described in any supporting publication. This is particularly important if strongly associated variables are candidates for inclusion. Further, if continuous variables are to be categorised, or categorical variables are to be reduced to binary form, then some justification for this should be provided.

In certain situations, there may be information from other research that a certain variable is of prognostic influence. In this case, the variable can be 'forced' into the model and this too should be reported. The subsequent selection procedure is then confined to the remainder of the variables.

Simon and Altman (1994) described the requirements necessary for studies which attempt to establish a particular measure or measures as prognostic. Of particular concern for them was to define clear phases in this process, analogous to Phases I, II and III used as stages of the development of a new drug in the clinical trial setting. They also provide valuable guidelines for the conduct and reporting of such studies. Their paper applies to all regression models and not just the Cox proportional hazards model described here.

8 | Time-dependent Variables

Summary

This chapter introduces 'time-dependent' explanatory variables or covariates, which are those whose value, for any given individual, may change over time. These are sometimes referred to as updated covariates. These contrast with covariates that remain fixed for all time for that individual. The Cox proportional hazards model can be extended to incorporate such variables. We present this extension and discuss the practical implementation of this methodology and subsequent interpretation of the results from such analyses.

8.1 INTRODUCTION

In the Cox models introduced in chapter 6 and developed in Chapter 7, we included only those covariates measured at a specific point in time, for example those recorded at the time of entry into a study, to help predict the future course of patients. Thus, in chapter 7 we considered whether a history of fits, patient age and tumour grade determined at the time of entry to the trial predicted the future course of patients with brain cancer. Thus at entry to the study—the single time point—a particular patient aged 40 may have a Grade 3 tumour but no prior history of fits. Such variables are known as 'fixed covariates' because they are observed or measured at a single point in time.

During the follow-up of patients, however, we will often obtain further information on some covariates which may, in fact, help us to better predict the subsequent course of the patient. For example, at a regular 3-month check-up of patients with brain cancer, the grade of the tumour may be reassessed. The now updated grade of the tumour at this 3-month check-up may then be a better indicator of future prognosis, as compared to the tumour grade recorded at entry into the trial. Biologically, one would anticipate that this may in fact be the case, since those patients with more aggressive disease at entry are likely to have a worsening tumour grade, indicating a progression of their disease. In contrast, those with less aggressive disease are more likely to have a static or even improving grade of disease at subsequent assessments following a period of treatment.

A further example of such a covariate is recurrent disease. Thus in patients with brain cancer, following surgical removal of their tumour, some may have a recurrence of their disease. Those experiencing a recurrence are likely to have a poorer subsequent prognosis than those remaining free of recurrence. Similarly, in a study of patients having received a heart transplantation, such as that described in section 1.1, patients may exhibit early signs of rejection. Such signs may give an early indication of poorer subsequent prognosis for the patient.

8.2 UPDATED COVARIATES

Such changing covariates are often known as 'time-dependent' covariates, in contrast to the 'fixed' covariates measured at a single point in time. Altman and de Stavola (1994) stress that the better phrase to use is 'updated covariates' since this emphasises that the value of the covariate is being updated with time.

They also make a useful distinction between *internal* and *external* variables. An example of an external variable is gender, which once observed remains fixed and unchanged. In contrast, an internal variable has the potential to change with time. Examples include blood pressure, which may be assessed at entry into a study, but has the potential to change thereafter, and tumour grade, which may or may not deteriorate with time. Clearly, changes in such internal characteristics can only be observed while the patient remains alive and will only be available for analysis if recorded.

We note that certain variables such as age, which although they change with time, are nevertheless deterministic and are in fact external covariates. This is because age, at any given follow-up time, can be completely predicted from the age at time of entry. However, even age could become an internal variable if it acts, for example, as a surrogate for menopausal status. For example, suppose menopausal status has not been recorded but age has, then women less than 45 years of age may be regarded, at least approximately, as premenopausal, those 45–55 as perimenopausal and those 55+ as postmenopausal. For such a variable, the states are not reversible. Thus, once postmenopausal status has been reached the woman cannot return to the premenopausal state. This contrasts with other examples in which a patient may pass in and out of various states as time passes.

Example

To illustrate both fixed and time-dependent covariates, Figure 8.1 shows the variation with time of anorexia symptom levels in three patients with small cell

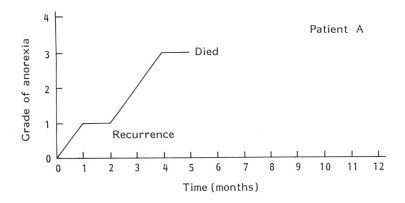

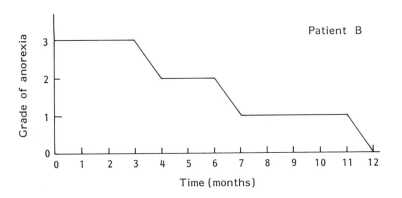

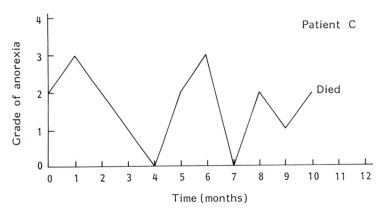

Figure 8.1 Profiles of anorexia symptom grade changes in three patients with small cell lung cancer (data from Medical Research Council Cancer Working Party, 1993, reproduced by permission of The Macmillan Press Ltd)

lung cancer. Loss of appetite in lung cancer patients may be an indicator of progressive disease. Those patients with no loss of appetite are scored anorexia grade 0, those with little loss, anorexia grade 1, those with 'quite a bit' of loss, anorexia grade 2, and those with substantial loss of appetite, grade 3. Thus, there are four possible states for these patients and, technically at least, a patient can move between any of them as time passes.

The grade of anorexia at presentation, which may be a summary of loss of appetite over a period prior to diagnosis, can be regarded as a fixed covariate. It therefore summarises the patient at that fixed point in time. As such it describes prognosis before commencement of treatment. Thereafter, the patient may show signs of further loss of appetite or may regain appetite depending on their response to treatment. This in turn may result in a gain or loss of weight. Thus, successive assessments of anorexia grade are values of an ordered categorical time-dependent or internal covariate.

Patient A, in the upper panel of Figure 8.1, presents with no evidence of anorexia; however, over the next 4 months the grade of anorexia steadily increases to the highest grade 3 corresponding to substantial loss of appetite, and the patient dies 1 month later. This patient had a recurrence of the disease at 2 months.

In contrast, patient B starts with a maximum grade 3 level of anorexia, but over a period of 12 months this steadily reduces, until follow-up at 1 year when the patient has no symptoms of anorexia at all. The patient has therefore essentially returned to his or her normal appetite before lung cancer took its toll. This patient is alive and free of recurrence at the 12-month time point. In such a patient the gradually reducing level of anorexia may be indicative of an improving prognosis.

Finally, patient C, in the lower panel of Figure 8.1, has a highly fluctuating level of anorexia, starting at level 2 and taking the minimum value at 4 and 7 months and the maximum value at 1 and 6 months. This patient died 10 months from entry to the study, with no recurrence of disease.

For illustrative purposes, the data points in Figure 8.1 are plotted at monthly intervals along the time axis, and therefore represent a somewhat idealised situation in which all patients are observed at regular (equal) intervals and their appetites assessed at that time. Even recurrence and death occurred at these convenient points! In reality, patients are assessed at somewhat irregular intervals, perhaps of approximately 1 month, and Table 8.1 gives the progress of 10 selected patients recruited to a lung cancer trial. Typically the date of entry to the trial is recorded, as well the anorexia grade (fixed covariate), on that occasion. The patient is then examined sometime later, when the date of visit and anorexia grade (time-dependent covariate) are again recorded. This process continues on a regular or irregular basis for each patient. In addition, the date of any recurrence of the disease is noted together with either the last date that the patient is known to be alive, or date of death if appropriate. These dates and anorexia symptom grades are included in Table 8.1.

From this table, it is then possible to calculate the day of successive visits relative to the date of entry to the trial. Similarly, time to recurrence and time of last follow-up or death are calculated for each patient. These are then collected together

Table 8.1 Progress of 10 patients with small cell lung cancer, giving anorexia grades at successive follow-up visits, date of recurrence and death

Patient number	Date of entry	Grade of anorexia	Date of visit 1	Grade of anorexia	Date of visit 2	Grade of anorexia	Date of visit 3	Grade of anorexia	Date of recurrence	Recurrence status 0 = Absent 1 = Present	Date of death/last follow-up	Survival status 0 = Alive 1 = Dead
1	18 Feb 85	0	11 Mar 85	0	1 Apr 85	0	09 Apr 85	0	14 Oct 85	1	27 Feb 86	1
2	06 Mar 85	3	02 Apr 85	0	23 Apr 85	–	16 May 85	0	29 Aug 85	0	29 Aug 85	1
3	21 Mar 85	2	09 Apr 85	3	30 Apr 85	2	21 May 85	1	10 Dec 85	1	10 Dec 85	0
4	28 Mar 85	1	13 May 85	2	04 Jun 85	1	07 Jun 85	2	29 Aug 85	1	02 Dec 85	1
5	03 Apr 85	0	25 Apr 85	0	16 May 85	1	28 May 85	1	23 Jul 85	1	06 Nov 85	1
6	17 Apr 85	0	13 May 85	0	05 Jun 85	0	03 Jul 85	0	05 Jun 85	1	16 Jan 86	1
7	13 May 85	0	13 Jun 85	0	01 Jul 85	0	–	–	29 Nov 85	1	16 May 87	1
8	05 Jun 85	0	26 Jun 85	0	17 Jul 85	0	29 Aug 85	2	19 Sep 85	0	31 Jan 86	0
9	18 Jul 85	2	13 Aug 85	2	–	–	–	–	13 Aug 85	0	13 Aug 85	0
10	13 Sep 85	1	–	–	–	–	–	–	10 Oct 85	0	31 Oct 85	1

Table 8.2 Progress of 10 patients with small cell lung cancer, giving anorexia grades at successive follow-up visits, time to recurrence and death, summarised from Table 8.1

Patient number	Initial anorexia grade	Time of visit 1 (days)	Grade of anorexia	Time of visit 2 (days)	Grade of anorexia	Time of visit 3 (days)	Grade of anorexia	Time of recurrence (days)	Recurrence status 0 = Absent 1 = Present	Time of death/last follow-up (days)	Survival status 0 = Alive 1 = Dead
1	0	21	0	42	0	50	0	238	1	374	1
2	3	27	0	48	–	71	0	176	0	176	1
3	2	19	3	40	2	61	1	264	1	264	0
4	1	46	2	68	1	71	2	154	1	249	1
5	0	22	0	43	1	55	3	111	1	217	1
6	0	26	0	49	0	77	0	77	1	274	1
7	0	31	0	49	0	–	–	200	1	733	1
8	0	21	0	42	0	85	2	106	0	240	0
9	2	26	2	48	–	–	–	48	0	48	0
10	1	27	–	–	–	–	–	48	0	69	1

into a data matrix for analysis. The necessary calculations for the data of Table 8.1 result in the entries for the corresponding patients given in Table 8.2.

From this table, we see that patient 1 had anorexia grade 0 at admission and thereafter also grade 0 at 21, 42 and 50 days later. The patient had a recurrence of the disease after 238 days and died just over a year from entry at 374 days. The first three visits of patient 2 were completed by 71 days but the grade of anorexia was not recorded at visit 2. This patient died after 176 days, but with no evidence of a recurrence. A recurrence of disease was noted in patient 3 after 264 days, which was also the date of the latest survival information on that patient.

Typically, observing time-dependent data in patients generates complex data sets similar to those of Table 8.1. These are then manipulated into a summary format similar to that of Table 8.2 for analysis.

Example from the literature

Mackie *et al.* (1991) investigate, in potentially fertile women receiving treatment for melanoma, the influence on their subsequent survival of whether or not they conceive during the treatment period which commences following diagnosis.

The time-dependent covariate, in this example, takes the states pregnant or not pregnant. This is a binary variable which takes a value 0 from the date of commencement of anti-melanoma therapy to the date of conception, and thereafter takes the value 1 until the baby is born and then returns to 0. For a woman who does not conceive at any time subsequent to the commencement of her treatment, the time-dependent covariate remains at 0. In this example, there are two states (pregnant, not pregnant), which are reversible. Thus a woman could, potentially at least, be not pregnant at commencement of treatment, become pregnant, give birth and hence be no longer pregnant, then conceive again and so on.

It should be noted that time-dependent or updated covariates can also exhibit the tendency to be censored and, therefore, remain unobserved. Thus, for example, in the patients summarised in Figure 8.1, in addition to the time-dependent covariate anorexia, we may also be interested in using the time-dependent variable recurrence, to predict subsequent length of survival. However, in patients B and C a recurrence was not observed. In patient B such a recurrence is still potentially observable, but for patient C, who died at 10 months free from recurrence, there is no such possibility.

8.3   THE TIME-DEPENDENT EXTENSION OF THE COX MODEL

The first step in extending the Cox model to time-dependent covariates is to examine equation (6.12) again. We reproduce it here, in slightly modified form, for convenience. Thus, the relative hazard is expressed by

$$h = \lambda(t)/\lambda_0(t) = \exp(\beta x). \qquad (8.1)$$

In this model, x is a fixed covariate and β is the corresponding regression coefficient which is to be estimated from the data. We here assume that the relative hazard does not vary with time, t, and that is why it does not appear on the right-hand side of equation (8.1).

If x is a binary variable, then we have shown in equation (6.7) that $HR = \exp(\beta)$ in such a situation. On the other hand, if x is a continuous variable then, by comparison with equation (6.16), $HR = \exp[\beta(x_1 - x_2)]$, where x_1 and x_2 are the values of the variable in the two groups to be compared.

In the 'time-dependent' situation we can have a covariate which itself now varies with time. Suppose we define this variable as $z(t)$, to indicate that the value may change with t. In the example presented above, $z(t)$ would be successive measures of the level of anorexia. Declining values of $z(t)$, in this case an ordered categorical variable, indicate favourable response to treatment.

We use the notation z for a time-dependent covariate to distinguish from x, a fixed covariate, to ease the explanation of the technique. Hence, for a single time-dependent covariate $z(t)$, in place of x in equation (8.1) we write

$$h(t) = \exp[\gamma z(t)]. \tag{8.2}$$

Here γ is the regression coefficient and corresponds to β used previously in equation (8.1). The form of equation (8.2) now indicates that the relative hazard, h, depends on t. That is, the relative hazard may change with time.

Example

In the MRC Lung Cancer Working Party (1993) trial, 458 eligible patients with small cell lung cancer were randomised to receive one of three treatment regimens. These were three cycles of a four-drug chemotherapy (ECMV3), six cycles of the same chemotherapy (ECMV6) or six cycles of a two-drug chemo-therapy (EI6). A primary aim of this trial was to assess the survival on the three treatment arms.

As is the case for many clinical trials, however, data on covariates were collected both at entry to the trial and during the follow-up of individual patients. The 'follow-up' information was collected before each cycle of treatment (every 3 weeks) and then monthly for the first 12 months, and subsequently at 3-month intervals. Thus, in trying to predict the changing prognosis of these patients we could use all information, the fixed covariates taken at entry and the time-dependent recorded at follow-ups. However, for ease of presentation we confine our analysis to the data arising from the first three follow-up visits only.

Table 8.3 shows the proportion of patients experiencing each level of anorexia at entry to the trial and at the first three subsequent follow-up visits. In the table, the column headed 'Missing data' implies that for the number of patients indicated there are no data available on anorexia symptoms for whatever reason. This may include, for example, failure to record the information during the visit, a patient missing a visit, or death. The proportion of patients with missing data increases as time increases. Thus, approximately 2% (10/458) of patients have missing data, concerning the level of anorexia, at entry to the trial, while by the third visit 35% (163/458) of patients have missing data on this variable. The percentage of missing data gradually increases over the three

Table 8.3 Level of anorexia symptoms recorded for 458 patients, with small cell lung cancer at successive visits. Percentages have been calculated of the total non-missing information at that visit (data from MRC Lung Cancer Working Party, 1993, reproduced by permission of The Macmillan Press Ltd).

Time point	Missing data	Level of anorexia							
		None (0)		Little (1)		Quite a bit (2)		Much (3)	
Pretreatment	10	220	49%	134	30%	79	18%	15	3%
Visit 1	68	233	60%	100	26%	50	13%	7	2%
Visit 2	84	242	65%	88	24%	38	10%	6	2%
Visit 3	163	210	71%	526	18%	26	9%	7	2%

visits. This is quite typical in follow-up studies of seriously ill patients but it does illustrate that obtaining complete data on time-dependent covariates can be a problem.

It is also of some interest to note that, if we look at the percentages in the four anorexia groups of these patients, we see that by the time of the third visit, there is an apparent increase in the proportion of patients with no anorexia symptoms. There is a corresponding reduction of patients with symptoms coded as 'little' or 'quite a bit' of anorexia. This trend may be a consequence of the treatment given, i.e. the treatment the patients are receiving is indeed reducing the level of anorexia. However, it is also possible that it is due to the fact that those with a higher level of anorexia symptoms are likely to have died by this time and consequently have become a disproportionate proportion of the 163 patients with 'missing data' at the third follow-up. This is very likely to be the case and so care needs to be taken in interpreting such time-dependent data.

8.4   BINARY VARIABLES

The simplest example of a time-dependent covariate is one that can only take two values. Thus we first consider anorexia symptoms as though it was a binary variable, i.e. it is either present or absent in each patient at the respective assessments. To create a binary variable for anorexia symptoms involves combining groups 1 (a little), 2 (quite a bit) and 3 (much) into a single group indicating presence of 'anorexia' (group 1) and comparing these patients with those with 'no anorexia' (group 0). In this way, we create a factor for anorexia having two levels which we denote by **An**. This factor can then be included in the modelling process. We denote the factor as **An** rather than **A** here to avoid confusion with models including age that we have described in earlier chapters.

FIXED COVARIATE ONLY

For comparison purposes we first establish a fixed covariate model, relating length of survival to presence or absence of anorexia, at entry to the trial. The fixed covariate Cox model takes the form

$$\textbf{An}: h = \exp(\beta x) \tag{8.3}$$

where $x = 0$ for patients with no anorexia, and $x = 1$ for patients with some anorexia at entry to the trial.

In fitting this model, we obtain an estimate for the fixed regression coefficient β as $b = 0.4525$, with a SE $= 0.0974$. The LR of this model, when compared to the null model, is $LR_{An,(1)} = 21.564$ with df $= 1$, which implies a p-value <0.001.

From this result we can say, since b is positive and statistically significant, that there is good evidence that patients with anorexia symptoms at entry to the trial have a poorer prognosis than those who do not. We conclude that having symptoms increases the risk of death by a factor of $HR_{Fixed} = \exp(0.4525) = 1.57$.

TIME-DEPENDENT COVARIATE ONLY

In the time-dependent covariate situation, equation (8.3) is replaced by

$$\textbf{An}(t): h(t) = \exp[\gamma z(t)]. \tag{8.4}$$

Anorexia is now a time-dependent factor which we have emphasised by use of $\textbf{An}(t)$ as our description of the model.

However, we now need to consider the form for $z(t)$. One possibility is to ask whether the current or latest information available on anorexia is indicative of survival. For example, it may be that those patients with a better prognosis transfer from 'some anorexia' to 'no anorexia' during the follow-up visits. In this case $z(t) = 0$ if there are no anorexia symptoms present at the last available data point and $z(t) = 1$ if anorexia symptoms are present at the last available data point. The bold entries in Table 8.2 indicate the data on anorexia grade used in such a time-dependent analysis. Thus for patients 1 to 6 and 8 the anorexia symptoms are those recorded at visit 3, for patient 7 the value is that of visit 2, for patient 9 that for visit 1 and for patient 10 the value is the pretreatment or initial anorexia grade. We recall that those patients with values of 2 and 3 are recoded as 1 for this binary variable example.

Fitting model $\textbf{An}(t)$ for all patients gives an estimate for the time-dependent regression coefficient, γ, as $c = 0.6154$, with a SE $= 0.0997$. The LR for the model, as compared to the null model, is $LR_{Time-Dependent} = 35.940$ with df $= 1$. This gives a p-value of <0.0001. Thus, there is good evidence to state that those patients with symptoms of anorexia recorded at their last data point have a poorer prognosis than those without anorexia.

However, the interpretation of the increased hazard associated with the presence of anorexia, which is expressed by $HR_{Time-Dependent} = \exp(0.6154) = 1.85$, is less straightforward. We have seen above that, in the fixed variable model, the regression coefficient represents the change in the hazard associated with having, or not having, anorexia symptoms at entry to the trial. In the time-dependent model, however, the coefficient reflects the increased hazard of having anorexia symptoms (as opposed to having no anorexia symptoms) at the *last point* that such information was available. As we have noted, this last information may in fact be the data collected at entry for some patients or at the third visit for others.

In the time-dependent model, we assume that the increased hazard associated with symptoms of anorexia is the same at whichever time it is observed. Thus, the increased hazard is the same irrespective of whether, for example, this observation was made at the end of the third visit or at entry to the trial. This means that in this model the effect is considered as independent of the timepoint at which the information is available for each patient.

There are also some practical difficulties, above and beyond those for fixed covariates, in assessing and interpreting the results of the time-dependent analysis of anorexia, especially in terms of 'cause and effect'. It may be that the presence or absence of anorexia at a given point in time is largely a reflection of the effect of treatment. A successful treatment may not only prolong life but, at the same time, reduce symptoms of anorexia. In this case, we may then observe a statistical association between length of survival and current symptoms of anorexia, but a 'cause and effect' relationship may not necessarily exist between them.

Altman and de Stavola (1994) describe practical problems in fitting a proportional hazards model to data from time-dependent covariates.

FIXED AND TIME-DEPENDENT COVARIATE MODEL

We next consider whether time-dependent, and therefore updated, information on anorexia symptoms adds useful prognostic information to that already available at entry. For example, in the most extreme case where no patient changed their status of anorexia symptoms over the first three visits, the updated information on anorexia exactly reproduces the information collected at entry. No additional information is therefore gained. We can assess the value of any extra information available by combining equations (8.3) and (8.4) into the following model:

$$\text{An} + \text{An}(t): h(t) = \exp[\beta x + \gamma z(t)]. \tag{8.5}$$

This model has both a fixed-covariate term and a time-dependent covariate term. The model can be formally tested using the methods introduced in chapter 7, to determine whether removing either the time-dependent or the fixed anorexia covariate significantly reduces the variation explained by the combined model. Table 8.4 shows the results of fitting both the fixed and time dependent variables separately and together. The table also includes the LRs obtained by comparing each of these models with the null model.

Comparing the LRs for the fixed covariate model, $LR_{An} = 21.564$, with that for the combined fixed and time-dependent model, $LR_{An + An(t)} = 50.944$, gives $LR_{Difference} = LR_{AN + An(t),An} = 50.944 - 21.564 = 29.38$. This comparison has df = 1 and associated p-value of <0.0000001, which is very strong evidence that the updated time-dependent anorexia symptoms variable contributes significantly to the combined model and that it would be unwise to ignore the information it provides.

Similarly, removing the fixed anorexia symptoms term gives $LR_{Difference} = LR_{An + An(t),An(t)} = 50.944 - 35.940 = 15.004$ with df = 1, giving a p-value ≈ 0.0001. This provides good evidence that the fixed anorexia variable adds significantly to the combined model and it would be also inappropriate to leave this variable out.

These results suggest, perhaps rather counterintuitively, that when used as binary

Table 8.4 Fixed and time-dependent models for binary anorexia symptoms, with associated regression coefficients and LRs, in patients with small cell lung cancer (data from Medical Research Council Lung Cancer Working Party, 1993, reproduced by permission of The Macmillan Press Ltd).

Anorexia model	Regression coefficient (b)	SE	Regression coefficient (c)	SE	LR	df	p-value
Fixed only, **An**	0.4525	0.0974	–	–	21.564	1	<0.0001
Time-dependent, **An**(t)	–	–	0.6154	0.0997	35.940	1	<0.0001
Fixed and time-dependent, **An** + **An**(t)	0.3804	0.0982	0.5599	0.1007	50.944	2	<0.0001

variables presence or absence of time-dependent anorexia and the pretreatment anorexia symptoms both provide useful and largely independent information on the subsequent length of patient survival. It is useful to note that this relative independence is supported by the fact that the regression coefficient estimates, given in Table 8.4, of the two-variable model, i.e. $b = 0.38$ and $c = 0.56$, are similar to those given in the corresponding single-variable models with $b = 0.45$ and $c = 0.62$. This is often a good indication of the independent behaviour of two variables in a model.

The final model is therefore written

$$\textbf{An} + \textbf{An}(t): h(t) = \exp\{0.38\,[\text{Pretreatment anorexia}] + 0.56\,[\text{Latest anorexia}](t)\}. \quad (8.6)$$

Here the t indicates the anorexia grade which was determined at the last available follow-up visit at which information was recorded.

Example from the literature

In the study reported by Mackie *et al.* (1991) in 388 women with melanoma they included the four fixed covariates, tumour thickness (continuous), site of disease (categorical of three groups), parity (ordered categorical of five values) and delivery (ordered categorical of three levels) as well as the time-dependent pregnancy status (binary) that we have indicated earlier, in a Cox model. They conclude that tumour thickness, site and parity are important prognostic variables for survival but the time-dependent pregnancy status is not.

The authors do not appear to state the number of events, here deaths, on which these conclusions are based but their survival curves suggest this may be only about one-quarter the number of patients or 100 deaths. If this is indeed the case, then there are probably too few events for such an analysis which required the estimation of 11 regression coefficients.

8.5 CATEGORICAL VARIABLES

We can extend the models specified in equations (8.3), (8.4) and (8.5) to categorical variables of $g(>2)$ groups. For example, if we now define anorexia symptoms as an

Table 8.5 Fixed and time-dependent models for anorexia treated as an ordered categorical variable, with associated regression coefficients and LRs, in patients with small cell lung cancer (data from Medical Research Council Lung Cancer Working Party, 1993, reproduced by permission of The Macmillan Press Ltd)

Anorexia model (ordered categorical variable)	Regression coefficient (b)	SE	Regression coefficient (c)	SE	LR	df	p-value
Fixed only: **An**	0.2793	0.0602	–	–	20.644	1	<0.0001
Time-dependent: **An**(t)	–	–	0.4275	0.0649	38.828	1	<0.0001
Fixed and time-dependent: **An** + **An**(t)	0.1875	0.0624	0.3658	0.0678	47.664	2	<0.0001

ordered categorical variable, with three levels—0 = none, 1 = a little and 2 = quite a bit or very much—then this three-level variable can be included in the modelling process. Note that from the data of Table 8.2 we have collapsed the original categories 2 and 3 into one category. This is necessary because, in our example, the proportion of patients in the 'very much' category is too small to allow sensible estimation of the corresponding regression coefficient.

Table 8.5 shows the results of fitting the fixed, and now ordered categorical variable with three levels, covariate anorexia model, the time-dependent ordered categorical covariate model for anorexia also of three levels, and finally the combined fixed and time-dependent model. We note that we are fitting these models with the categories given values 0, 1 and 2 and are not using the dummy variable technique.

The results of Table 8.5 show a similar picture to that of Table 8.4 when anorexia symptoms were reduced to a binary variable. In particular, both the time-dependent and fixed variables are separately useful in predicting length of survival. Further, omitting either variable from the model containing both variables, leads to a significant reduction in the variation explained by the model. The difference in LRs for leaving out the time-dependent variable is $LR_{Difference} = 47.664 - 20.644 = 27.020$ with df = 1. This gives a p-value <0.000001. The same difference for the fixed variable is $LR_{Difference} = 8.836$, again df = 1, giving a p-value of 0.003.

We should note that since both variables have ordered categories, then the estimated $HR_{An} = \exp(b) = \exp(0.2793) = 1.32$ and $HR_{An}(t) = \exp(c) = \exp(0.4275) = 1.53$ represent both the increased hazard of being in category 2 (quite a bit, substantial) rather than category 1 (a little) and the increased hazard of being in category 1 rather than category 0 (none).

If the time-dependent categorical variable has g categories that are not ordered then such a variable has to be fitted using g – 1 dummy variables as in the fixed-covariate case discussed in section 6.9. No new principles are involved.

8.6   CONTINUOUS VARIABLES

Continuous covariates can be handled in the same way as ordered categorical variables. As in the fixed covariate case, however, it is usual for the mean value of the time-dependent covariate to be subtracted from each data point to improve the stability of the calculation of the regression coefficients in the Cox model. It may also be useful to look at a plot of the data to assess approximate normality, although, as for the fixed-covariate case, variables included in the model do not have to be normally distributed. It may be an aid to numerical stability in the calculation procedure to transform covariates, which have skewed distributions, perhaps using a logarithmic transformation to obtain a more symmetric distribution shape.

Example from the literature

Fisher *et al.* (1991) investigate the influence of the time-dependent covariate ipsilateral breast tumour recurrence (IBTR), as a predictor of the development of distant tumour in women who had had a lumpectomy following diagnosis of breast cancer. We discussed aspects of the fixed-covariate part of this model in section 6.9.

The results of their Cox regression model are summarised in Table 8.6. The risk associated with IBTR is summarised by $HR_{IBTR(t)} = 3.41$ with a 95% CI of 2.70 to 4.30. We have included (t) in the HR term to indicate a time-dependent covariate has been modelled. The authors conclude from this analysis that the patients' expected risk of developing distant disease is greater once an IBTR is evident. For some women in the study, no IBTR was diagnosed and so their expected risk for a distant

Table 8.6 Cox regression model using fixed and time-dependent covariates as predictors of time to distant disease in 1000 patients with breast cancer (From Fisher *et al.*, 1991, Significance of ipsilateral breast tumour recurrence after lumpectomy, *Lancet*, 338, 327–331, © by The Lancet Ltd)

Covariate	Regression coefficient	SE	χ^2	p-value	HR(95% CI)
Fixed					
Age (years)	0.257	0.108	5.79	0.016	1.29(1.05–1.60)
Nodal status					
Absent	0	–			
Present	0.433	0.107	16.20	0.0001	1.54(1.25–1.90)
Nuclear grade					
Low	0	–			
High	0.399	0.111	13.01	0.0003	1.49(1.20–1.85)
Tumour type					
Good	0	–			
Intermediate	0.544	0.209	7.67	0.0056	1.72(1.14–2.60)
Poor	0.751	0.215	14.15	0.0002	2.12(1.39–3.23)
Time-dependent					
IBTR	1.226	0.119	88.06	<0.0001	3.41(2.70–4.30)

tumour is based solely on their personal and tumour characteristics noted at the initial operation. As a consequence, their prognosis is based on fixed covariates.

It is of further interest to note that the authors do not consider there to be a 'casual' link. This is because the appearance of the IBTR is most likely a 'marker' for an unknown risk factor already present. In theory, if we knew this marker we would not then need the knowledge of whether or not there was an IBTR.

Example from the literature

Farewell (1979) investigates the relation between the time to appearance of an infection, using a time-dependent analysis of data arising from a randomised trial of laminar airflow (LAF), in patients with aplastic anaemia and acute leukaemia, receiving bone marrow transplants (BMT). In this trial, 89 patients were randomised following BMT, either to a LAF isolation room or to usual patient care.

The aim was to assess whether the protective environment of the LAF room (the 'treatment' variable) decreases the infection rate once an allowance for any other factors influencing risk of infection had been made. In addition to treatment (LAF or no LAF), the four fixed covariates recorded at entry to the trial were age, marrow cell dose, sex match of the donor, and whether or not recipient infections prior to transplantation were recorded. The two time-dependent covariates were the occurrence of graft versus host disease (GVHD) and granulocyte level post BMT, as these were also thought to influence a patient's risk of infection. GVHD is a binary variable and granulocyte count a continuous variable.

Farewell reports an analysis including only four of these variables. These were the 'treatment' allocated, the fixed covariate of evidence of prior infection and the two time-dependent covariates GVHD and granulocyte count. This analysis is summarised in Table 8.7.

Table 8.7 Prediction of time to infection in 89 patients with aplastic anaemia and acute leukaemia using Cox's time-dependent covariate model (From Farewell, 1979. Reproduced by permission of the Royal Statistical Society)

Covariate		Value	Regression coefficient	SE	HR	p-value
Fixed						
T: LAF room	x_T	No	0	–	1	
		Yes	−0.909	0.346	0.403	0.008
I: Prior infection	x_I	No	0	–	1	
		Yes	−0.183	0.627	0.833	0.780
Time-dependent						
G(t): GVHD	$z_G(t)$	No	0	–	1	
		Yes	−0.225	0.773	0.799	0.780
LGr(t): log (granulocyte count)	$z_C(t)$		−0.151	0.086	0.860	0.080

The fixed covariate—prior infection—is clearly a binary variable taking the value 1 when a prior infection had been observed and 0 otherwise. Thus the values of the fixed covariates are $x_T = 1$ if the patient is allocated to the LAF room and $x_T = 0$ if not, together with $x_I = 1$ if prior infection is recorded and $x_I = 0$ if not. The time-dependent covariate GVHD occurs as an immunological reaction of the new marrow graft against the patient. This was defined as a binary variable with a value of 0 if no GVHD exists and the value 1 after GVHD occurs. It is also well established that the granulocyte count is of major importance in determining a patient's susceptibility to infection. Following transplantation, a patient's granulocyte level is expected to fall rapidly and then gradually to return to a normal level. This variable was recorded on a daily basis for all patients on study and the log (granulocyte count) rather than the count itself was used as a time-dependent variable in the proportional hazards model. The values of the time-dependent covariates are therefore $z_G(t) = 1$ if GVHD occurs and $z_G(t) = 0$ if it does not, and $z_C(t) = $ log (granulocyte count).

In this situation, the time-dependent Cox model can be specified as

$$T + I + G(t) + LGr(t): h(t) = \exp\{\beta_T x_T + \beta_I x_I + \gamma_G z_G(t) + \gamma_C \log [z_C(t)]\}. \quad (8.7)$$

Here β_T and β_I are the regression coefficients for the fixed covariates of treatment and infection, and γ_G and γ_C are the regression coefficients for the time-dependent covariates.

The only two important factors resulting from this analysis appear to be treatment, with use of the LAF room having an associated $HR_T = 0.4$, (p-value = 0.008) and granulocyte count. The latter indicates that for every log (granulocyte count) reduced by 1 unit, for example from 1000 to 368 since log $1000 = 6.9$ and log $368 = 5.9$, there is a reduced $HR_{Gran(t)} = 0.86$ (p-value = 0.080). The author states that although granulocyte count appears of only marginal conventional significance, since the p-value = 0.08 is greater than 0.05, it should be retained in the model because earlier studies had established its relationship to infection.

8.7   CHOOSING THE 'BEST' MODEL

The choice of which covariates, whether fixed or time-dependent, to include in a model follows the same processes as described for the fixed variable models in chapter 7. In this process, time-dependent variables are treated in the same manner as fixed variables.

One particular problem with time-dependent covariates is the multiplicity of variables available for analysis. For example, with the anorexia symptom data, instead of considering the last available value of anorexia, we could have considered the difference between this value and the value at entry as our variable, or equally possible the maximum value over visits. The first of these investigates whether it is the change in grade of symptom score with time that is important for prognosis. The latter asks if it is the worst grade of anorexia which is predictive of subsequent survival. It is quite plausible that any, or all, of the variables defined in this way will help to predict the future course of patients. When we multiply these possibilities by the number of variables available we can see that it will often be possible to specify numerous time-dependent covariates which can be included in the model. Thus, by chance alone, some will be 'significantly' related to survival. In this context we have to be even more aware that validation of any model, preferably using an independent dataset, is required.

8.8 CHECKING THE ASSUMPTION OF PROPORTIONAL HAZARDS

We discussed the use of the complementary logarithmic plot to verify if the hazards corresponding to different values of a particular fixed covariate are proportional in section 6.13. An alternative approach to assessing proportionality for a fixed covariate, essentially extends the fixed-covariate model for variable x, described by equation (8.1), to that of the time-dependent equation (8.5), with a special format for $z(t)$. In the case where the fixed covariate is a binary variable taking values $x = 0$ or 1, this special format is

$$z(t) = \gamma xt. \tag{8.8}$$

This then gives the a variables, one fixed the other time-dependent, model as

$$h(t) = \exp(\beta x + \gamma xt). \tag{8.9}$$

In equation (8.9) if $x = 0$ then $\gamma xt = 0$ also and the relative hazard is now not dependent on time, t. In contrast, when $x = 1$ we have $\gamma xt = \gamma t$, and the relative hazard is clearly dependent on t except in the special situation that $\gamma = 0$.

For this model with two groups, the HR is the ratio of equation (8.9) evaluated at $x = 1$ and $x = 0$. Thus

$$HR(t) = \exp(\beta + \gamma t)/\exp(0) = \exp(\beta + \gamma t) \tag{8.10}$$

since $\exp(0) = 1$. In this situation the HR is clearly a function of time except in the special case when $\gamma = 0$. Finally, equation (8.10) can be expressed as

$$HR(t) = \exp(\beta)\exp(\gamma t). \tag{8.11}$$

This is the product of the HR obtained from the fixed-covariate model of equation (8.1) and $\exp(\gamma t)$, which depends on time.

Thus, if we fit equation (8.9) to our data and then test the hypothesis that the regression coefficient, γ, for the time-dependent covariate, t, which is time itself, is zero, we are testing the departure from proportional hazards in the two fixed-covariate groups corresponding to $x = 0$ and $x = 1$.

If, as a result of the test we can indeed conclude that $\gamma = 0$, then equation (8.11) implies that $HR(t) = HR$ and, therefore, is independent of time. In these circumstances we conclude the hazards are proportional.

In contrast, if following the test we conclude $\gamma \neq 0$ then the corresponding HR depends on time and the hazards are not proportional. In this model, if the HR increases over time, then γ will be estimated to be greater than zero, while if the HR decreases over time γ will be estimated to be less than zero.

The same idea can be extended to detect departure from proportional hazards in ordered categorical data of more than two levels. Thus for an ordered categorical or a continuous fixed covariate, say y, we can fit the model

$$HR(t) = \exp(\beta y + \gamma y t). \qquad (8.12)$$

As previously we test whether the coefficient γ is significantly different from zero. Again, an estimate of $\gamma < 0$ suggests a decreasing HR with time, while an estimate of $\gamma > 0$ suggests an increasing HR, as compared to a convenient reference value of y. This is often taken as its mean value if the variable is continuous.

<table>
<tr><td>9</td><td>Prognostic Indices</td></tr>
</table>

Summary

This chapter describes how to use a Cox model to determine a prognostic index to help classify patients into different risk groups. Discussion of which patient variables to include and how the risk groups are formed and used is presented. We stress the roles of training and confirmatory data sets, respectively, to establish and verify the prognostic index. Finally, we include a description of how a well-established prognostic index may be updated.

9.1 INTRODUCTION

As we have seen, one important application of the Cox's proportional hazards model is to help identify variables which may be of prognostic importance. Once identified, knowledge from these may be combined and used to define a prognostic index, which in turn defines groups of individuals at differing risk. To use the prognostic index, key patient characteristics are recorded at diagnosis and from these a score is derived. This score gives an indication of whether, for example, the particular patient has a good, intermediate or bad prognosis for the disease.

9.2 SELECTING A MODEL

From the data of a randomised trial of misonidazole plus radiotherapy versus radiotherapy alone for patients with cancer of the brain, conducted by the MRC Working Party on Misonidazole in Gliomas (1983), and discussed in chapter 7, a Cox's proportional hazards model was used to identify a set of variables influencing the duration of survival of these patients. In particular, we identified in

Table 7.4 that the two variables, age and length of history of fits, were useful in helping to predict the duration of survival in these patients.

In a complete analysis conducted by the MRC Brain Tumour Working Party (1990), four variables were identified that collectively were useful in predicting the length of survival. These were age (A), categorised as <45, 45–59, ≥60 years; clinical performance status (C), categorised as 0–1, 2, 3–4; extent of neurosurgery (N), categorised as complete, partial, biopsy only; and length of history of fits (F), categorised as ≥3 months, <3 months, none. This last categorisation contrasts with our previous analysis in chapter 7, which categorised patients as either having or not having a history of fits. It is useful to note here that we have ordered the categories, in a sense, from good to bad with respect to prognosis. Our knowledge of the disease suggests this order to us. This choice helps the interpretation as, if we are indeed correct, then the corresponding regression coefficients should all be positive and the HRs will be greater than 1. Also in this analysis, the three category levels of each factor were coded 0, 1 and 2 and treated as a continuous variable measured on this three-point scale. By assigning the values 0, 1, 2 to each of the categories, this implicitly means that one is assuming a linear trend in survival across each factor. In particular that the patient group with value 0 has the best prognosis, the group with value 1 has intermediate prognosis, while the group with value 2 has the worst prognosis. We do not know if the corresponding regression coefficients are statistically significant until we fit and test the models.

The authors used both forward and backward variable selection procedures, as described in chapter 7, with both procedures identifying these same four factors as the important variables. All other recorded variables were taken as not adding further prognostic information.

Table 9.1 Prognostic factors and prognostic index scores derived from 417 patients with brain cancer (data from Medical Research Council Brain Tumour Working Party, 1990)

Prognostic factor	Category	Category score	Estimated coefficient (b)	SE(b)	HR	Index score
Age (A)	<45	0	0	–	1	0
	45–59	1	0.3366	0.0719	1.40	7
	≥60	2	0.6732		1.96	14
Clinical performance status (C)	0–1	0	0	–	1	0
	2	1	0.2084	0.0594	1.23	4
	3–4	2	0.4168		1.52	8
Extent of neurosurgery (N)	Complete	0	0	–	1	0
	Partial	1	0.2279	0.0693	1.26	5
	Biopsy only	2	0.4558		1.58	10
Length of history of fits (F)	≥3 months	0	0	–	1	0
	<3 months	1	0.2434	0.0714	1.28	5
	None	2	0.4868		1.63	10

The final form of the Cox model calculated from data for the 417 patients with brain tumours was

$$\textbf{A} + \textbf{C} + \textbf{N} + \textbf{F}: h = \exp(\beta_A A + \beta_C C + \beta_N N + \beta_F F). \tag{9.1}$$

The estimates of the regression coefficients of equation (9.1) are $b_A = 0.3366$, $b_C = 0.2084$, $b_N = 0.2279$ and $b_F = 0.2434$. These, together with the associated SEs and HRs for each level of these prognostic factors, are given in Table 9.1. For example, for patients who are 45–59 years of age, $HR = \exp(0.3366 \times 1) = \exp(0.3366) = 1.40$, whilst for those aged ≥ 60 the $HR = \exp(0.3366 \times 2) = \exp(0.6732) = 1.96$. Both these HRs are expressed relative to those patients of <45 years.

9.3   DEVISING A PROGNOSTIC INDEX

Once a model has been established, to develop a prognostic index (PI) for use with future patients it is necessary to calculate the value of equation (9.1) for each of the 417 patients in the trial. This is done using values for their individual categories, as set out in Table 9.1. These are based on patient characteristics at a medical examination at the time of diagnosis of their tumour. Thus, for example, a patient at presentation, aged 63 (Category score 2), with clinical performance status 2 (Category score 1), having complete neurosurgery (Category score 0) and no experience of fits (Category score 2), will have from equation (9.1) a relative hazard of

$$h = \exp(0.3366 \times 2 + 0.2084 \times 1 + 0.2279 \times 0 + 0.2434 \times 2)$$
$$= \exp(1.3684) = 3.929. \tag{9.2}$$

For convenience, rather than using h as the score for each patient, we use log h, which is in effect the exponent part of equation (9.1) or equation (9.2). Thus, for the above patient the score, S, is now

$$S = \log h = 1.3684. \tag{9.3}$$

In a similar way, a patient less than 45 years old, with a clinical performance status of 2, having a partial resection and no history of fits, has the following score:

$$S = 0.3366 \times 0 + 0.2084 \times 1 + 0.2279 \times 1 + 0.2434 \times 2$$
$$= 0.9231$$

This calculation is then repeated for the remaining 415 patients in the trial. Since there are four factors each of three possible values, or levels, there are theoretically $3^4 = 81$ different scores possible. These range in value from $S = 0$, for patients less than 45 years, clinical performance 0 or 1, complete neurosurgery and a history of fits of duration in excess of 3 months, to $S = 2.0326$ for patients aged 60 years or more with clinical performance status 3 or 4, biopsy only and no history of fits.

The frequency distribution of the 417 resulting scores is given in Figure 9.1 and shows that the majority of patients have scores between 0.7 and 1.7. There are relatively few patients with very low scores: only two patients with $S < 0.1$; but quite a few with very high scores: 26 patients with $S \geq 2.0$.

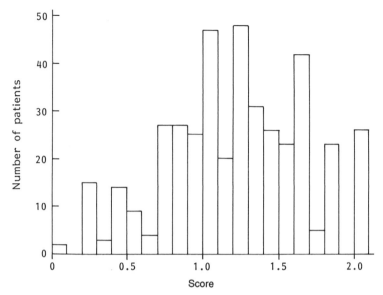

Figure 9.1 Grouped frequency distribution of scores derived from a Cox model fitted to the survival information of 417 patients with brain cancer (data from Medical Research Council Brain Tumour Working Party, 1990)

The next step, at least in theory, is to calculate the separate Kaplan–Meier survival curves for the resulting 81 score groups. However, in this example, there are clearly too few patients per group for this purpose, since there will be an average of only 5 ($417/81 = 5.15$) patients per group. In point of fact, there are fewer than 81 distinct groups as some of the 3^4 combinations result in the same score. Neither would it be sensible to calculate the survival curves of patients in the 19 groups of Figure 9.1 as again there are too few patients in some of these groups. Instead, we first partition the scores into convenient, often arithmetically convenient, groups with sufficient patients per group. For example, we might identify patients with low scores ($S < 1$), medium scores ($1.0 \leq S < 1.5$) and high scores ($S \geq 1.5$). We then calculate the corresponding survival curves calculated from the individual patients falling into these three groups. In our example, the low, medium and high score groups have 126, 172 and 119 patients, respectively. The corresponding survival curves are shown in Figure 9.2. These show the rather better outcome for the low score (better risk) patients, who have a median survival time of approximately 1 year. This contrasts with, for example, the poor risk group, who have a median survival of approximately 4 months.

As one might expect, the survival curves also indicate a gradient of survival differences between the three score groups.

To derive a PI, which can be used more easily than calculating the rather difficult score, S, it is usual to simplify the regression coefficients in the fitted Cox model of equation (9.1). One way of doing this is as follows: we begin with the exponent part of the fitted Cox model

$$S = 0.3366A + 0.2084C + 0.2279N + 0.2434F. \tag{9.4}$$

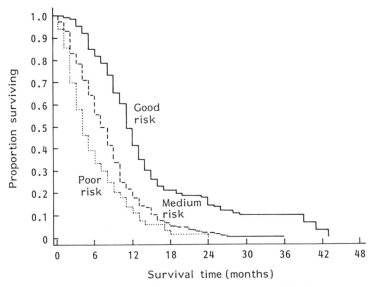

Figure 9.2 Kaplan–Meier survival curves for low, medium and high score groups derived from 417 patients with brain cancer (data from Medical Research Council Brain Tumour Working Party, 1990)

We note the regression coefficients are in the ratio 3366 : 2084 : 2279 : 2434. The decimal place in equation (9.4) is of no consequence here since the same multiplicative change in all the regression coefficients affects all patients and hence preserves their rank order with respect to their values of S. This ratio is, after multiplying the coefficients by 2, approximately 67 : 42 : 46 : 49, which, in turn, is very similar to 70 : 40 : 50 : 50 or finally 7 : 4 : 5 : 5! There is a balance here between strictly preserving the ratios of the regression coefficients as they appear in equation (9.4), while at the same time arriving at modified coefficients that are easy to work with. That is, they are both arithmetically simple to manipulate and easy to remember. Once derived, these modified coefficients are used to replace the score S of equation (9.4) by the PI. This is given by the equation

$$PI = 7A + 4C + 5N + 5F. \tag{9.5}$$

As a consequence, we replace, for the patient who is aged 63, clinical performance status 2, having complete neurosurgery and no history of fits, the score $S = 1.3684$ by $PI = (7 \times 2) + (4 \times 1) + (5 \times 0) + (5 \times 2) = 28$. Similarly for the patient with $S = 0.9231$ we have $PI = (7 \times 0) + (4 \times 1) + (5 \times 1) + (5 \times 2) = 19$, and so on for the remaining 415 patients.

Alternatively, the patient characteristics can be identified against the entries in Table 9.1 and the corresponding index scores in the final column noted. The PI for each patient is then just a sum of the appropriate four index scores.

The PI can be calculated for each of the 417 patients in the study, and not surprisingly the shape of the resulting frequency distribution of the individual PI's is similar to that for the score S shown in Figure 9.1. The values of the PI range from 0 to 42, corresponding to S equal to 0 and 2.0326, respectively. A high score of the PI indicates a worse prognosis than a low one.

Finally, the distribution of the PI is examined and convenient subgroups of differing prognosis are identified. We choose three convenient groups as 0–19, 20–29 and 30–42 for this purpose. The boundaries of the risk groups, i.e. 20 and 30, are first chosen here for convenience of memory. Table 9.2 shows the number of patients in each of the groups, together with the corresponding median survival times and the Kaplan–Meier 2-year survival rates. The corresponding survival curves of the patients divided into these three groups, classified as good, medium and poor risk patients, are shown in Figure 9.3.

There are minor differences in the patients selected to each PI group from those of Figure 9.2, but these are most likely in patients with scores close to the boundaries of the respective risk groups. Thus, there are 111 patients in the good

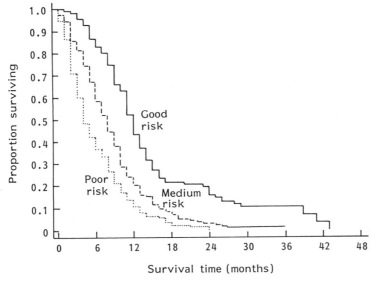

Figure 9.3 Survival curves for the three patient groups identified on the basis of a prognostic index (data from Medical Research Council Brain Tumour Working Party, 1990)

Table 9.2 Number of patients, median and 2-year survival according to prognostic group for 417 patients with brain cancer (data from Medical Research Council Brain Tumour Working Party, 1990)

Prognostic index	Risk group	Number of patients	Median survival (months)	2-year survival
0–19	Good	111 (27%)	12	16%
20–29	Medium	161 (39%)	8	3%
30–42	Poor	145 (35%)	4	0%

risk group of Table 9.2 (PI of 0–19), in contrast to 126 with good risk as classified by S<1. This is due to both the modified regression coefficients used in the calculations and to changes in the relative positions of the convenient boundaries chosen to define the good, intermediate and poor risk patients.

Example from the literature

Leonard *et al.* (1991) present a PI for low-grade non-Hodgkin's lymphoma, derived from survival information on 506 patients. Their PI requires information on ECOG performance status, age, stage of disease, sex and haemoglobin levels at presentation. This is summarised in Table 9.3.

This PI includes the continuous variable haemoglobin which is treated as such in the Cox model. Thus, although very simple scores are attached to performance status, age, stage and sex, and these are easily summed, it is also necessary to subtract the score for haemoglobin. This makes the calculation of the final PI somewhat less straightforward.

Examples of three patients with non-Hodgkin's lymphoma are given by the authors and the characteristics of these are summarised in the final columns of Table 9.3 against the corresponding variable category and associated component score contributing to the PI. The score for patient A is, therefore, $1 + 0 + 1 + 0 + (-0.27 \times 13) = 2 - 3.51 = -1.51$.

In this example, those with a negative score (patient A) are regarded as having the best prognosis, those with a score between 0 and 3 (patient B) intermediate

Table 9.3 Relevant presentation features and scores for three patients with non-Hodgkin's lymphoma (From Leonard *et al.*, 1991. Reprinted by permission of Kluwer Academic Publishers)

Presentation feature	Category	Score	Patient A	Patient B	Patient C
ECOG performance status	0	0			
	1 or 2	1	ECOG 2	ECOG 2	ECOG 1
	3	2			
	4	4			
Age (years)	≤49	0	49 years		
	50–65	2		65 years	
	66+	4			66 years
Stage	1	0			
	2, 3 or 4	1	Stage 4	Stage 3	Stage 2
Sex	Female	0	Female	Female	
	Male	1			Male
Haemoglobin	g/dl	−0.27	13 g/dl	12 g/dl	10 g/dl
		Score	−1.51	+0.76	+4.30

prognosis and those with a score ≥ 3 (patient C) as the worst prognosis group. It is then easy to remember that a negative PI suggests the best prognosis and a PI of 3 or more the worst. Use of haemoglobin as a continuous variable, in this way, has the advantage of not introducing rather artificial break points for this variable, above which a patient is of good prognosis, below which, bad. However, it does have the drawback of being more cumbersome and less easy to remember.

It is worth noting that the groups derived by Leonard *et al.* (1991) were established on the basis of those 25% (lower quartile) with the worst prognosis, the intermediate 50% and finally 25% (upper quartile) with good prognosis. This approach guarantees sufficient patient numbers in the risk groups, but does not necessarily give convenient boundaries.

9.4 TESTING THE PROGNOSTIC INDEX

The PI developed for the brain tumour patients provided good discrimination between poor, medium and good risk groups. However, as we have used the same data to develop the PI, often called the training set, it is hardly surprising that we observe such good discrimination between the risk groups. In short, we cannot use a single set of training data both to develop and test a PI. To test the PI appropriately we need an independent or confirmatory data set.

For our example, a confirmatory data set is provided by a subsequent MRC multi-centre trial of two doses of radiotherapy in patients with cancer of the brain (Bleehen and Stenning, 1991) in which stage, age, performance status and duration of history of fits were also recorded. In this (second) trial, patients with brain tumours of either Grade 3 or 4 astrocytoma were randomised to receive either 45 or 60 Gy of radiotherapy treatment.

Using the information from these patients, the earlier derived PI of equation (9.5) was used to score each patient. The patients were then placed in the appropriate risk groups, defined with boundaries at 20 and 30, respectively, as previously specified. The survival curves for the three prognostic groups for these 'confirmatory' patients are shown in Figure 9.4.

It can be seen from Figure 9.4 that, although there is still a clear distinction between 'good', 'medium' and 'poor' risk groups, the separation between the three confirmatory data groups is not quite as marked as that of Figure 9.2. In particular, the medium and poor risk groups have 'shrunk' closer to each other, although the good risk group appears to have a relatively, but small, improved prognosis. These differences are no more than we might expect because the PI is unlikely to provide such a good separation between groups in an independent data set, as was observed in the data set used to derive it. The 'shrinkage' is, in fact, a well-known phenomenon that is often observed in confirmatory data sets.

Table 9.4 shows the percentage of patients in each risk group together with the associated median and 2-year survival figures, and when compared to Table 9.2, confirms slight 'shrinkage' of the medium and poor risk groups indicated by Figure 9.4, the corresponding estimates of median survival now being 9 and 6 months, respectively (ratio 1.5, difference 3), as compared with 8 and 4 months (ratio 2.0, difference 4) in the training data set. However, both these groups and the

Table 9.4 Number of 'confirmatory' patients in each prognostic group and survival in each prognostic group for patients with astrocytoma (data from Bleehen and Stenning, 1991, reproduced by permission of The Macmillan Press Ltd)

Prognostic index score	Risk group	Number of patients	Median survival (months)	2-year survival (%)
0–19	Good	92 (21%)	14	28
20–29	Medium	175 (39%)	9	9
30–38	Poor	176 (40%)	6	2

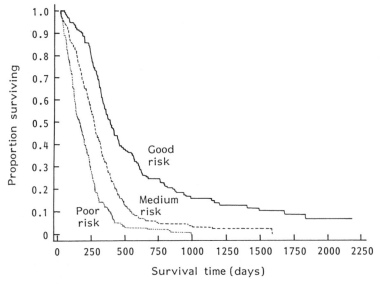

Figure 9.4 Survival curves of good, medium and poor prognosis groups of patients with astrocytoma (data from Bleehen and Stenning, 1991)

corresponding good risk group appear to have a better survival than those of Table 9.2, from which the PI was derived. Nevertheless, the separation between the three groups remains good and we have, therefore, confirmed the value of the PI.

Example from the literature

Leonard *et al.* (1991) in deriving their PI for patients with low-grade non-Hodgkin's lymphoma, which is given in Table 9.3, first divided the 506 patients into two data sets. The training set consisted of 326 patients, from which a PI was derived. This PI was then tested on the second or confirmatory data set, which comprised 180 patients recruited from a geographically distinct area of the Edinburgh and Border regions of Scotland. The survival curves of these 180 patients, divided into best, intermediate and worst prognostic groups on the basis of the score calculated from

Table 9.3, is shown in Figure 9.5. The authors conclude that the PI they derived from the training set does indeed discriminate well between the three risk groups so established.

We have indicated some necessary steps required when constructing a PI. The aim of such an index is to identify patients with differing risk. It must be remembered that the divisions established for the risk groups are in some sense arbitrary, so that even within a PI group there may be substantial variation in prognosis.

Prior to easy access to powerful and inexpensive personal computers, emphasis was placed in deriving a PI that was very easy to compute and the boundaries of the 'at risk' groups easy to define. Thus, arithmetically simple and memory-jogging numbers were often used in the PI. However, it may now be relatively easy to write a menu-driven computer program that can calculate a PI directly from, for example, equation (9.2) or equivalently the regression coefficients in Table 9.1. The

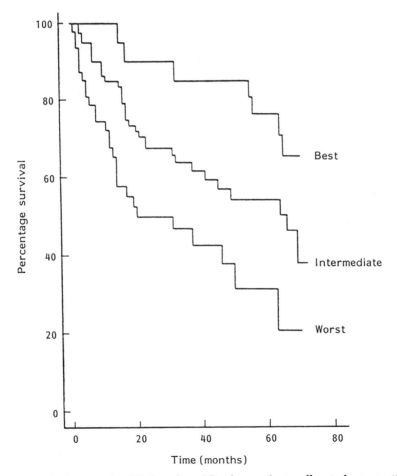

Figure 9.5 Survival curves for Edinburgh and Borders patients, allocated prognostic groups on the basis of a prognostic index (From Leonard *et al.*, 1991. Reprinted by permission of Kluwer Academic Publishers)

examining clinician merely records the patient details and feeds them to the program, which then returns the PI group and associated risk for that patient.

9.5   THE ROLE OF TREATMENT

In developing the PI with the brain tumour patients, a regression coefficient to account for the treatment received by the patient was not included in the model of equation (9.1). This was because no survival difference between patients allocated to the two treatments was observed. However, for the patients of the confirmatory data set, a survival difference between the two treatments allocated was observed. The results reported by Bleehen and Stenning (1991) gave an HR = 0.81 for survival, with 95% CI of 0.66 to 0.99, in favour of the high dose regimen. This difference obviously accounts for some of the variability observed, in that those patients who receive the 'better' treatment have on average a better survival time. In this context, it is of interest to assess whether the PI appears relevant to patients in both treatment groups. Figure 9.6(a) shows the survival curves by prognostic group for those patients allocated to receive a low-dose radiotherapy of 45 Gy and Figure 9.6(b) shows the same for those allocated to receive a high-dose radiotherapy of 60 Gy.

It can be seen that the separation between the three prognostic groups is maintained in both treatment groups. It is a common experience that, in many cases, prognostic factors are often independent of the treatment given. However, we should note that although the separation between the groups remain, the actual curves for the individual groups receiving the two treatments may differ. For example, the survival for the good risk group who receive 60 Gy is likely to be higher than for the same good risk group but who receive 45 Gy. This is confirmed by Figure 9.6(a,b).

When the data to develop a PI come from a randomised trial, the differing treatments are well defined and can be included in the model with ease. In contrast, if the data arise from, say, a retrospectively inspected series of case records, there

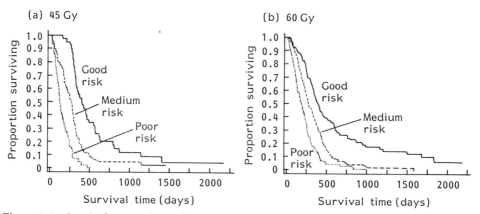

Figure 9.6   Survival curves for each prognostic risk group by treatment allocated in patients with astrocytoma (data from Bleehen and Stenning, 1991, reproduced by permission of The Macmillan Press Ltd)

may be many different treatments employed. To take account of these, we would need either to add many terms to the model by use of dummy variables or attempt to summarise the numerous possibilities into broad treatment groupings. In the latter case, we may, for example, classify the treatments into broad categories of chemotherapy, radiotherapy or surgery. Once summarised in this way, treatment could then be added to the models for developing the PI.

9.6 UPDATING THE PROGNOSTIC INDEX

Once the PI has been tested on a confirmatory data set, it may be appropriate to refine and update the index by pooling the data from both sets. In such cases, it is usually not sensible to begin the model selection process all over again, since we have, at least in our example, firmly established the four important prognostic factors. What we do instead is to fit these factors to the combined dataset and thereby obtain modified estimates of the corresponding regression coefficients. A new and updated PI will be derived from these.

However, there are two further aspects that have to be considered. First, there may be a significant survival difference observed between the treatments. Second, if we are combining data from two or more trials, then the type of treatments used may differ and it is possible that the magnitude of the effect of a prognostic factor may also differ, depending on the treatment.

Consider again the example of patients with brain tumours. To allow for the treatment effect, we incorporate a term for treatment, T, into the Cox model of equation (9.1) as follows:

$$T + A + C + N + F: h = \exp(\beta_T T + \beta_A A + \beta_C C + \beta_N N + \beta_F F) \qquad (9.6)$$

For brevity, we have indicated in equation (9.6) that only one regression coefficient, β_T, is needed in order to include the effect of treatment in the model. In fact, how the treatment effect is included in the model will depend on the treatment-specific features of the training and confirmatory data sets. For example, for the data from the two trials in patients with brain tumours, the patients of the training data received either placebo or misonidazole in addition to radiotherapy, while those of the confirmatory data received radiotherapy at doses of either 45 or 60 Gy. In this situation, we can describe the effect of treatment in three different ways in the model of equation (9.6) and which are summarised in Table 9.5.

In the first method, the four different treatments are regarded as such and, therefore, can be classified as four levels of a non-ordered categorical variable. This can then be incorporated into equation (9.6) using the three dummy variables g_1, g_2, g_3. This is referred to as Model I in Table 9.5. Each of the three dummy variables will have an associated regression coefficient γ_1, γ_2 and γ_3. The estimates of these are given as c_1, c_2 and c_3 in the second (updated) column of Table 9.6.

Comparing these results with those of Table 9.1, which are reproduced in the 'original' column in Table 9.6, we see that the regression coefficient for age has increased somewhat, from 0.3366 to 0.4678. In contrast, the coefficient for extent of neurosurgery has become smaller, from 0.2279 to 0.1571. The regression coefficients

Table 9.5 Models for including treatment in the development of a prognostic index for patients with brain tumours

Data set	Treatment	Model I			Treatment	Model II	
		g_1	g_2	g_3		g_4	g_5
Training	Placebo	0	0	0	Control	0	0
	Misonidazole	1	0	0	Test	0	1
Confirmatory	45 Gy	0	1	0	Control	1	0
	60 Gy	0	0	1	Test	1	1

Table 9.6 Fitting Model I of Table 9.5, together with the confirmed prognostic variables from an earlier analysis, to the combined data of two randomised trials in patients with brain tumours (data from Bleehen and Stenning, 1991, reproduced by permission of The Macmillan Press Ltd)

Factor		Estimated regression coefficients		
		Original (from Table 9.1)	Updated	SE
Treatment				
Placebo		–	0	–
Misonidazole	c_1	–	−0.1959	0.0954
45 Gy	c_2	–	−0.0919	0.1079
60 Gy	c_3	–	−0.3558	0.0898
Prognostic variables				
A	b_A	0.3366	0.4678	0.0500
C	b_C	0.2084	0.2403	0.0436
N	b_N	0.2279	0.1571	0.0471
F	b_F	0.2434	0.2411	0.0487

for clinical performance status and length of history of fits have stayed largely unchanged. This suggests that, by including the patients from the confirmatory data set into the model, age has become a more important prognostic factor, while the extent of neurosurgery has become less important. Following these changes in the estimates of the regression coefficients through, by the process described in section 9.3, results in an updated PI of the form

$$PI(updated) = 9A + 5C + 3N + 5F. \tag{9.7}$$

We note that the PI does not contain terms associated with the effect of treatment, despite treatment being included in the model. This is because treatment was included in the model only to obtain adjusted estimates of the coefficients of the PI. When the PI is used for future patients, the treatment employed is chosen, and may in fact be different from those used in the patients in our examples. The four other variables, however, are fixed for each patient at the time of diagnosis.

This updated PI implies, in broad terms, that age is now approximately twice as important as clinical performance status and length of history of fits, and three times as important as the extent of neurosurgery. Previously in the PI of equation (9.5) there was less variation in the weights attached to the prognostic factors.

Two further aspects should be noted in Table 9.5. First, the SEs for the estimates are smaller than in Table 9.1. This is because the number of deaths available for this analysis is approximately double that of the earlier analysis. Second, the estimate for the treatment effect has no straightforward interpretation. Note, however, that fitting treatment-specific coefficients will, in general, also contribute to smaller SEs for the regression coefficients of each prognostic factor.

Model II of Table 9.5 recognises explicitly that there are two data sets a and a and models this with $g_4 = 0$ and 1, respectively, with associated regression coefficient γ_4. Control and test therapies within these data sets are then modelled with $g_5 = 0$ and 1 respectively, with associated regression coefficient γ_5. Fitting this model to the data gives estimates of these regression coefficients as -0.1317 and -0.2268 respectively. More importantly, for our example, the corresponding estimates for the regression coefficients for age, clinical performance status, extent of neurosurgery and length of history of fits of 0.4670, 0.2411, 0.1571 and 0.2421 differ very little from those of Model I, summarised in Table 9.6. As a result, the updated PI with this form of the model remains as equation (9.7).

A third possible model to include the effect of treatment in the process of updating the PI adds a treatment by data set interaction term to Model II. This Model III replaces the term $\gamma_4 g_4 + \gamma_5 g_5$ in Model II by $\gamma_4 g_4 + \gamma_5 g_5 + \gamma_{45} g_4 g_5$, the latter representing the interaction term. Fitting this model to the data gives estimates of these regression coefficients as -0.1599, -0.2638 and 0.0679 respectively. The first two of these are very close to the values of -0.1317 and -0.2268 for the corresponding Model II values and the coefficient for the interaction term is close to zero. More importantly for our application, however, the regression coefficients for age, clinical performance status, extent of neurosurgery and length of history of fits of 0.4678, 0.2408, 0.1571 and 0.2411, respectively, are very close to those of Model II. As a result, the updated PI with this model again remains as equation (9.7).

Although there is little or no difference in the updated PI derived from Models I, II or III, this will not always be the case in other examples. In such situations, some care must then be taken in choosing the final model for the PI.

9.7   TESTING AN ESTABLISHED PROGNOSTIC INDEX

In certain circumstances, a PI is so well established that to change it on the basis of new information may not be very practicable. Clearly if the new information suggests that the very basis of the PI needs to be questioned, then that is a different matter. Suppose that the PI is indeed well established, implying that the model from which it derives is also well established, both in terms of the variables it contains and also the value of the corresponding regression coefficients. To establish if the new information is going to influence the estimates of the regression coefficients, one can use the procedure described in the following example.

We assume our model includes only age and history of fits and is of the form $\mathbf{A} + \mathbf{F}$ of equation (7.6). Thus $h = \exp(S) = \exp(0.6528x_A - 0.4647x_F)$. We now wish to determine if we need to modify the estimates of the regression coefficients of this model with our new data. The procedure is first to calculate the score, S, for all the new patients. We then fit the model

$$h = \exp(S + \beta_{SA}x_A + \beta_{SF}x_F) \tag{9.8}$$

to our data. Here, β_{SA} and β_{SF}, represent the extra information in the new data on the influence of age and history of fits on prognosis.

We now test the null hypotheses for the regression coefficients, i.e. $\beta_{SF} = 0$ and $\beta_{SA} = 0$. If both these hypotheses are not rejected, the model remains that of equation (7.6). This implies that the regression coefficients for calculating S remain unchanged. On the other hand, if either of the null hypotheses is rejected, then the corresponding regression coefficients in S are modified by adding the estimates of β_{SA}, β_{SF} or both, to b_A and b_F as appropriate. Such a change or changes are then carried through to the PI, which may or may not be affected depending on the magnitude of these changes in the regression coefficients.

If the possibility of adding a single new variable, v, is under consideration, then equation (9.8) is modified to

$$h = \exp(S + \beta_v v). \tag{9.9}$$

In this case, the null hypothesis of $\beta_v = 0$ is tested. Once more, if the null hypothesis is not rejected, then the model S is not modified. On the other hand, if the hypothesis is rejected, then S is updated by addition of the new variable, v. This will clearly affect the PI, perhaps in a substantial way.

If both modifications to existing regression coefficients and the possibility of new variables are being considered then equations like (9.8) and (9.9) can be combined in an obvious way. Special procedures have to be used to fit models (9.8) and (9.9). These procedures essentially force the model both to give S a regression coefficient of 1 (S can be written $1 \times S$) and also to keep the variable S in the model if a selection procedure for the other variables is used.

10 | Sample Sizes for Survival Studies

Summary

This chapter describes how sample sizes can be determined for survival studies comparing the survival curves of two treatment groups. To obtain such sample sizes, it is necessary to specify at the planning stage of the study the size of the effect that is anticipated together with the size and power of the test to be used for the comparison. Formulae and tables for logrank comparisons are provided. We stress the approximate nature of sample size calculations and indicate that proposed studies with inadequate power should be considered carefully before their implementation.

10.1 INTRODUCTION

One important problem to address once the design of a particular study has been decided is an appropriate sample size. A study that is too small may not be able to answer the question posed; one that is too large will be wasteful of resources. We have given several examples in earlier chapters of clinical trials in which patients are recruited and randomised to receive a particular treatment, then followed up until a critical event occurs. An associated survival time for each patient is then used to compare the Kaplan–Meier estimates of the respective survival curves. The relative efficacy of the two treatments is then tested, using the logrank test described in chapter 4. We have emphasised that it is not essential that all patients must be followed until the critical event occurs. Indeed, in many situations this is not possible as, for example, in cancer trials some patients may survive many years after randomisation and it is thus not practicable to await their death before analysis. Nevertheless, as we have seen, such a patient is used in the treatment comparison, although the event of interest has not been observed. The sample size calculations we describe do therefore incorporate censored data.

To illustrate the sample size calculations, we will assume that we are planning a clinical trial of two alternative therapies, and that the design team are aware of the results of a preliminary trial and will use this information for planning purposes. We should also note that preliminary or 'first' trials often give 'overestimates' of the effect size which is subsequently observed in a (usually larger) confirmatory trial. It should also be emphasised that the randomised trial is only being used here as one of many possible illustrations.

To assist in the description of sample size calculations, we use the notation indicated in Figure 10.1, which shows two exponential survival curves. Each of these are of the form illustrated in Figure 3.1. There is one curve corresponding to the survival of patients receiving standard or control treatment, C, and one for those receiving the new or test treatment, T. Although we are concerned with survival time studies using the HR as the associated summary statistic, one often uses survival rates at particular (fixed) times for planning purposes, because they are often easier to specify. Further, as we shall see, these fixed time point survival rates can be translated into a HR.

The number of subjects necessary to recruit to a particular clinical trial depends on several factors. These include: the anticipated difference between the treatments, often termed the effect size; the level of statistical significance required; and the power or chance of detecting the effect size postulated.

In addition we need to specify the shape of the relationship between the two survival curves. For this we consider two possibilities: one in which survival curves are assumed to follow exponential distributions; and the other, less restrictive, assumption in which the hazards for the two groups are merely assumed to be proportional.

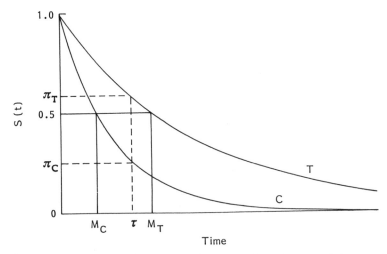

Figure 10.1 Anticipated exponential survival curves of patients receiving control, C, and test, T, therapies for a particular disease

Example from the literature

Valerius *et al.* (1991) described a small trial of 26 patients with cystic fibrosis who were randomised to receive either no treatment or anti-pseudomonas treatment for *Ps. aeruginosa* in their sputum. In this trial, 12 patients were randomised to no treatment (control) and the remaining 14 to anti-pseudomonas treatment. The 'survival' time recorded in this case is the time that the patients' sputum is free of colonisation by *Ps. aeruginosa*, as measured from the date of randomisation to the first positive test of their sputum.

The results are shown in Figure 10.2, which gives the approximate colonisation-free rates at 12 months as $p_C = 50\%$ for the untreated patients and $p_T = 85\%$ for those receiving treatment. This difference can be expressed as an observed advantage to the treated group of $p_T - p_C = 35\%$ at 1 year. However, with such a small trial there inevitably remains considerable uncertainty surrounding this outcome.

In the simplest case we use this trial as providing basic planning information for a further trial addressing the same question. The preliminary trial suggests an improvement in colonisation-free rates with the treatment, T, of 35% at 1 year over a colonisation-free rate of 50% with control, C. If these results are then expressed in the notation of Figure 10.1, $\tau = 1$ year, and the anticipated colonisation-free rate for C is $\pi_C = 0.5$ and that anticipated for T is $\pi_T = 0.85$. We note that we replace the observed p_T and p_C by π_T and π_C, respectively, to indicate that the latter are now the assumed values which we use for planning purposes. However, for the confirmatory trial we will also assume that there remains considerable scepticism

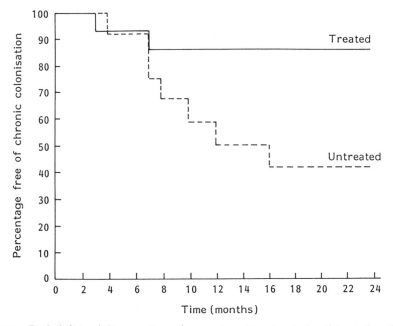

Figure 10.2 Probability of *Ps. aeruginosa*-free sputum in untreated and treated patients with cystic fibrosis (From Valerius *et al.*, 1991, Prevention of chronic *Pseudomonas aeruginosa* colonisation in cystic fibrosis by early treatment, *Lancet* 338, 725–726, © by The Lancet Ltd)

about the positive nature of the preliminary trial results and that there still remains a possibility that the anti-pseudomonas therapy may have an adverse effect on outcome.

Theory, formulae and tables for the calculation of sample sizes for the logrank test are given by Machin and Campbell (1987). There are also computer programs available for this purpose.

10.2   DEFINING EFFECT SIZE

SURVIVAL AT A FIXED TIME POINT

Figure 10.1 shows that at some fixed time τ the proportion of patients alive is $S_T(\tau) = \pi_T$ for the test treatment and $S_C(\tau) = \pi_C$ for the control. In this illustration, the proportion remaining alive at any time is greater in those patients who have received T as compared to those who have received C. If we assume that the survival curves have an exponential distribution, then we have from equation (3.3)

$$\pi_T = S_T(\tau) = \exp(-\lambda_T \tau) \tag{10.1}$$

where λ_T is the constant hazard for treatment T. We can rewrite equation (10.1) as

$$\lambda_T = -\log \pi_T / \tau. \tag{10.2}$$

In a similar way, we obtain for the control group at the same time τ

$$\lambda_C = -\log \pi_C / \tau. \tag{10.3}$$

As a consequence, the ratio of the two hazards, which determines the corresponding anticipated HR for summarising the difference between the two treatment groups, is

$$\frac{\lambda_T}{\lambda_C} = \frac{\log \pi_T}{\log \pi_C} = \Delta. \tag{10.4}$$

We denote the HR in equation (10.4) as Δ rather than HR since Δ is specified before the start of the trial, while HR is estimated at the end of the trial. Here we interpret Δ as the anticipated value of the HR, i.e. the true underlying HR, which we wish to estimate with the data from our clinical trial that we are now planning. The null hypothesis, H_0, states that the true value of the HR is unity, which will be the case if there is truly no difference in survival in the two treatment groups (see section 1.4). The value Δ provides us with the anticipated value of the HR under the alternative hypothesis, often denoted by H_A.

Example

We assume the colonisation-free times in the two treatment groups of the trial of Valerius et al. (1991) both have an exponential distribution with different but constant hazards. In that case, at $\tau = 1$ year, with an anticipated colonisation-free rate, $\pi_T = 0.85$, and use of equation (10.2) gives an anticipated hazard

$\lambda_T = -\log \pi_T/\tau = -\log(0.85)/1 = -(-0.1625)/1 = 0.1625$ for patients receiving T. In a similar way, the anticipated hazard for treatment C is $\lambda_C = -\log(0.50)/1 = -(-0.6931)/1 = 0.6931$.

As a consequence, equation (10.4) gives the anticipated HR as $\Delta = \lambda_T/\lambda_C = 0.1625/0.6931 = 0.23$. This suggests an HR of developing infection for those patients receiving active therapy of approximately one-quarter of that for those remaining untreated.

We note that the anticipated effect size can be expressed as either $\delta = \pi_T - \pi_C = 0.85 - 0.50 = 0.35$ as we indicated earlier, or as $\Delta = 0.23$. On these two scales the null hypothesis of no treatment effect is expressed either by $\delta_0 = 0$ or $\Delta_0 = 1$, respectively. The subscript 0 reminds us that these are the effect sizes anticipated by the null hypothesis.

MEDIAN SURVIVAL

In some situations it is more natural to think of anticipated differences in terms of a difference in median survival times, rather than in terms of a difference in survival rates at a particular fixed timepoint. However, for exponentially distributed survival times, there is a direct relationship between the median survival and the survival rate observed at a fixed time.

Suppose the anticipated median survival time for one of the treatment groups is M. By definition, the proportion surviving to the median time is 0.5 and so $\exp(-\lambda M) = 0.5$. This in turn gives, using equation (10.2), the hazard

$$\lambda = -\log 0.5/M. \tag{10.5}$$

In our example we can then substitute the anticipated median survival times for treatments C and T in equation (10.5) in turn to obtain the corresponding values for λ_C and λ_T. These lead to the anticipated HR of equation (10.4) as

$$\Delta = \frac{\lambda_T}{\lambda_C} = \frac{M_C}{M_T}. \tag{10.6}$$

Thus Δ is merely the inverse of the ratio of the corresponding median survival times for treatments T and C. Therefore, at the planning stage of a trial we can calculate the anticipated hazard ratio Δ, either from the proportions expected to be alive with each treatment at a fixed time, or from the respective median survival times.

Example

For those patients on control the median colonisation-free time in the example of Figure 10.2 is approximately 1 year. In this case, equation (10.5) gives $\lambda_C = -\log 0.5/1 = 0.6931$. By coincidence this is exactly the same value as we obtained using the fixed time point method to obtain the control group hazard since the median and fixed time point chosen coincide at 1 year.

In general, the two approaches will provide similar estimates of the hazard if the survival does indeed follow an exponential distribution. However, in our example, had we chosen the fixed time point as 18 months or 1.5 years, as opposed to 1 year, then Figure 10.2 suggests $\pi_C = 0.40$ which leads to $\lambda_C = -\log 0.4/1.5 = 0.6109$ rather than 0.6931. Such a disparity suggests that some care needs to be taken in the choice of the fixed time point used for estimating survival rates. In general, it is advisable to take values which are close to the median survival time. It is also important to recognise that the width of confidence intervals surrounding the Kaplan–Meier estimates of the survival curve increases as we move to the right along the survival curve. Thus estimates of the anticipated hazard obtained from fixed time points in such regions may be very imprecise.

We cannot estimate the median colonisation-free time for the treated group of Figure 10.2. This is because the Kaplan–Meier estimate for that group remains above 50% for the 24 months reported. As a consequence the median survival method of equation (10.6) cannot be used to define the anticipated HR.

To obtain an anticipated HR as large as that observed using the 1-year time points, i.e. $\Delta = 0.23$, the median colonisation-free time with anti-pseudomonas therapy would need to be approximately 4 years.

In some circumstances, although one may have an estimate of the control therapy π_C it may not be possible to obtain π_T as there have been, for example, no published survival curves using this therapy. In planning a trial in such a situation one may postulate directly a value for Δ, in which case it is useful to note that equation (10.4) can be rearranged to give

$$\pi_T = \exp(\log \pi_C/\Delta). \tag{10.7}$$

This expression can then be used to determine the anticipated survival rate, π_T, for treatment T, if values for π_C and Δ are provided.

PROPORTIONAL HAZARDS

Although the formulae given in equations (10.4) and (10.6) defining the anticipated effect size have been derived specifically for the case of two exponential survival distributions, they also apply in the more general situation when only proportional hazards are assumed. This enables them to be used for planning purposes in this wider context.

10.3 TEST SIZE

For design purposes, we first postulate a null hypothesis that there really is no difference between treatment and control. Thus, for the above example, we postulate that patients with cystic fibrosis experience chronic colonisation by *Ps. aeruginosa* at the same rate, irrespective of whether or not they receive treatment. As already indicated, this null hypothesis can be expressed as either $\delta_0 = 0$ or equivalently as $\Delta_0 = 1$. The latter is obtained by setting $\pi_C = \pi_T$ in equation (10.4), or equivalently $M_C = M_T$ in equation (10.6).

Now, even if this null hypothesis is actually true, i.e. there is truly no difference between treatment and control, we may observe at the conclusion of our new trial a value of the HR which is not exactly equal to 1. Under the assumption of no difference this will only be a random departure from the underlying $\Delta_0 = 1$. In this instance the difference between the observed HR and the value 1 will be due to chance alone and the associated p-value will not be small. On the other hand, if the p-value is small we are led to question whether the null hypothesis is indeed true. In fact, if the p-value is small enough we may reject the null hypothesis and conclude that the two treatments actually differ in their efficacy. This is equivalent to concluding that $\Delta \neq 1$.

When designing a trial, we have to decide at what level this p-value (probability) should be set, such that if a smaller p-value is observed we would reject the null hypothesis. The value we set at the design stage for this probability is often termed the test size and is denoted by α. It is also called the significance level or type I error. It is important to distinguish α from the p-value. The former denotes, at the planning stage, our pre-specified design significance level, while the latter is calculated at the analysis stage once our trial is completed. At this latter stage, if we observe a p-value $\leq \alpha$ then we reject the null hypothesis of equal treatment efficacy and conclude that the treatments do indeed differ in their relative efficacy.

Another way of viewing α is that it is the probability of falsely rejecting the null hypothesis. That is, if there is in truth no difference between treatment and control, it is our design probability that we will actually claim a difference between the two.

Although the choice of α is arbitrary, it has become common to set it at either 0.05 (5%) or 0.01 (1%), just as we commonly use either 95% or 99% confidence intervals.

10.4 POWER

Once we have specified the anticipated effect size, Δ, we need to ensure that the trial we have designed has a high probability of detecting this benefit should it, in fact, be the true underlying effect size. This probability is called the power of the study. Consequently, we require a small probability of our trial missing this benefit should it, in truth, exist. This small probability, β, is often called the false negative probability or the type II error. The power of study is $(1 - \beta)$ and is usually expressed as a percentage. In randomised trials the power is typically demanded to be high, for example at least 80% and quite commonly 90%.

Example

In planning the repeat of the randomised trial of Valerius et al. (1991), we may set an anticipated difference of $\Delta = 0.23$ and a power of $1 - \beta = 0.8$ or 80%. This design requires that if an underlying effect of $\Delta = 0.23$ is indeed present, then the new trial will have a good (80%) chance of reaching a statistically significant result at a pre-specified test size.

Although we have specified for this new trial that the anticipated benefit, derived from the earlier experience, is $\Delta = 0.23$, we have also indicated that this is a very large effect. If the design team are sceptical of this size of benefit truly existing, they may postulate an effect somewhat smaller than this, but which if demonstrated would still be important (see section 1.5). For example, they may think that $\Delta = 0.5$ or $1/2$ is more realistic than 0.23. In this case, they may prefer to design their trial with this alternative hypothesis in mind. In general, the closer the value of Δ is to the null hypothesis value $\Delta_0 = 1$, the larger the trial will need to be.

10.5 LOGRANK COMPARISONS ASSUMING PROPORTIONAL HAZARDS

EQUAL ALLOCATION

In many clinical trials, equal numbers of patients are randomised to receive one of two treatment options. A survival time for these patients is then observed and the treatments compared using the logrank test. As we have indicated, some patients may not experience the event of interest during their period of observation and so they will have censored survival times. The power of the study, and the width of the associated confidence interval for the observed HR, depends only on the number of events observed and not on the number of patients recruited. In some situations, for example lung cancer, patients die very quickly and death (the event) is then usually observed in most, if not all, patients within a reasonable time frame. In contrast, with a less aggressive disease, such as early breast cancer, the number of events observed in a reasonable time frame may be far less than the number of patients recruited.

It can be shown that if equal numbers of patients are allocated to each treatment, the total number of events, E, that need to be observed in a clinical trial comparing two treatment groups, with an anticipated benefit of Δ, test size α and power $1 - \beta$, is given approximately by

$$E = [(z_{1-\alpha/2} + z_{1-\beta})(1 + \Delta)/(1 - \Delta)]^2. \tag{10.8}$$

The terms $z_{1-\alpha/2}$ and $z_{1-\beta}$ are defined in section 1.2, and specific values corresponding to α and β are obtained from either Table T1 or T2 of the Normal distribution.

Example

For our example of patients with cystic fibrosis, we have indicated values for $\Delta = 0.23$, $\alpha = 0.05$ and $1 - \beta = 0.80$. Use of the two-sided column of Table T2 with $\alpha = 0.05$ gives $z_{0.975} = 1.96$ and use of the one-sided column with $\beta = 0.20$ gives $z_{0.8} = 0.8416$. Substituting these and $\Delta = 0.23$ in equation (10.8) gives $E = [(1.96 + 0.8416)(1 + 0.23)/(1 - 0.23)]^2 = 4.4753^2 = 20.03$ events.

This implies that we need to observe approximately 20 events to be reasonably sure to establish a benefit as extreme as $\Delta = 0.23$. That is, we would need to observe colonisation in at least 20 of the patients that we recruit to the proposed trial.

For the actual trial conducted by Valerius et al. (1991) this number of events implies that, for an effect size of $\Delta = 0.23$, colonisation needs to have been observed in 20/26 or 75% of the patients recruited. This was clearly not the case in the data reported in Figure 10.2 and suggests either that the trial was of insufficient size or had been reported too early.

ONE-SIDED AND TWO-SIDED TESTING

When designing a trial it is necessary to state whether a one-sided or two-sided test is going to be performed at the analysis stage. The decision depends upon the alternatives considered possible at the design stage. If we consider that there is a possibility the treatment may be worse than the control, although we anticipate it will be better, then we allow the possibility that the difference Δ can be greater than 1 (treatment worse) as well as less than 1 (treatment better). This situation would lead to a two-sided test being performed.

In fact, in most instances we are performing an experiment because we do not know whether the treatment is better, and there is usually a possibility (however small) that the treatment is worse. Thus a two-sided test is most often used. In rare circumstances it may be decided *a priori* that there is no possibility that the treatment is worse than the control. In this case the only alternative to the null hypothesis $\Delta = 1$, is that $\Delta < 1$ and a one-sided test would be performed.

Since one-sided tests are rare, the design formulae presented here assume a two-sided test will be performed. To adapt expression (10.8) to allow for one-sided testing merely involves replacing $z_{1-\alpha/2}$ by $z_{1-\alpha}$. For example, if we set our test size, α, to be 0.05 then a two-sided test would give $z_{1-\alpha/2} = 1.96$, while $z_{1-\alpha} = 1.6445$, leading to a smaller value of E for the one-sided test design. This will mean that a one-sided test design will always require fewer events to be observed than a two-sided test design.

It should be noted that a one-sided test should not be performed at the end of a trial which has been designed with a two-sided test in mind. Such an approach leads to a halving of the resulting p-value and may lead to results which are conventionally 'non-significant' (perhaps the two-sided p-value is greater than 0.05 but less than 0.1) being 'made significant' (one-sided p-value < 0.05).

Example

Gerhartz *et al.* (1993), in planning a randomised trial in patients with malignant non-Hodgkin's lymphoma, postulated an anticipated infection rate of 45% and 25% for the control and test therapies, respectively. They anticipated that the test therapy could only do better than the standard and hence would have fewer associated infections. In addition, they set $\alpha = 0.05$ and $1 - \beta = 0.8$.

By specifically excluding an adverse effect of therapy, although still stating the null hypothesis as $\Delta_0 = 1$, these investigators imply that the alternative hypothesis is $\Delta > 1$. This is a one-sided test situation and, as we have indicated, leads to replacing $z_{1-\alpha/2}$ by $z_{1-\alpha}$ in equation (10.8). Thus, we use the one-sided column of Table T2, rather than the two-sided column to obtain the corresponding value of z.

We first have to convert the infection rates into a 'success' rate, i.e. infection-free rates, just as we consider survival rates rather than mortality rates, to define the anticipated HR. Thus, the anticipated infection-free rates are 55% and 75% for the control and test treatments, respectively. The anticipated HR, $\Delta = \log 0.55/ \log 0.75 = 0.481$. Choosing a one-sided $\alpha = 0.05$, gives $z_{0.95} = 1.6445$ and a power of 80% gives $z_{0.8} = 0.8416$, from Table T2. Using these values in equation (10.8) gives the required number of events to be observed, $E = 50.3$. This implies that sufficient patients need to be recruited and randomised in equal numbers to each treatment option, in order to permit a total of approximately 50 infections to be observed.

If a two-sided, rather than one-sided test is to be performed then $\alpha = 0.05$, but $z_{1-\alpha/2} = z_{0.975} = 1.96$, from Table T2. The remaining terms retain their previous values. Using these values in equation (10.8) gives the required number of events, $E = 63.6$. Thus if a two-sided test is to be performed, then sufficient patients need to be recruited and randomised in equal numbers to each treatment option, in order to permit a total of approximately 64 infections to be observed. This is 14 more events than if a one-sided test is to be performed.

NUMBER OF SUBJECTS

It should be noted that equation (10.8) contains the benefit as expressed by the single summary Δ and gives the total number of events required, E. For this calculation, it is only necessary to specify the ratio of the treatment and control survivals, i.e. π_T/π_C, or alternatively the corresponding medians. However, in order to calculate the number of subjects required for the number of events, E, to be observed, it is necessary to specify their actual values. The total number of subjects required is then given by

$$n = 2E/(2 - \pi_T - \pi_C). \tag{10.9}$$

It is clear that this requires both the anticipated values π_C and π_T to be provided.

Example

Previous examples have shown for the trial of Valerius et al. (1991) that, if we were to repeat the trial using an anticipated HR of $\Delta = 0.23$, a two-sided $\alpha = 0.05$ (5%) and power $1 - \beta = 0.8$ (80%) then $E = 20.03$ events need to be observed. Their trial also indicated $\pi_T = 0.85$ and $\pi_C = 0.5$ and so the required number of patients, from equation (10.9), is $n = 2 \times 20.03/(2 - 0.85 - 0.5) = 40.06/0.65 = 61.6$. This implies that approximately 62 patients should be recruited to the confirmatory trial. Once these patients have been recruited then the analysis can take place once a total of 20 events has been observed.

To calculate the number of subjects required directly, equations (10.8) and (10.9) can be combined into a single expression to give

$$n = 2\left[\frac{(z_{1-\alpha/2} + z_{1-\beta})(1 + \Delta)}{(1 - \Delta)}\right]^2 \bigg/ (2 - \pi_T - \pi_C). \tag{10.10}$$

This combined expression is tabulated in Table T4 for a two-sided $\alpha = 0.05$, $1 - \beta$ of 0.8 and 0.9, a range of values of π_C ranging from 0.05 to 0.9 and the anticipated difference $\delta = \pi_T - \pi_C$ ranging from 0.05 to 0.5. Differences in the number of patients provided by direct use of equation (10.10) and Table T4 arise from roundings both in the calculations themselves and the final tabular entry, which is always rounded up to the nearest even number since we have assumed throughout two patient groups of equal size.

Example

For two-sided $\alpha = 0.05$, $1 - \beta = 0.8$, $\pi_C = 0.5$, $\delta = \pi_T - \pi_C = 0.85 - 0.50 = 0.35$, Table T4 indicates that $n = 66$ patients should be recruited. If we increase the power to $1 - \beta = 0.9$, then the number of patients required also increases, in this case, to $n = 88$. Thus, a randomised trial of 100 patients, 50 in each treatment group, may be appropriate in this situation.

PRACTICAL USE OF SAMPLE SIZE CALCULATIONS

Sample size calculations play an essential part in the design of any study. However, it must be recognised that there are a number of assumptions and 'guesstimates' which go into the calculation of the required sample size.

In particular in equation (10.10), although there are commonly accepted values for the test size, α, and the power $1 - \beta$, there is often considerable uncertainty over the values of π_C and π_T. Equivalently, we can say there may be considerable uncertainty over the values of π_C, and $\delta = \pi_T - \pi_C$. Table T4 shows how the numbers of subjects required varies for different values of π_C and δ and with the power. From this table we can see that small changes in δ can have an enormous impact on the number of subjects required. For example, if we set $\pi_C = 0.45$, $\alpha = 0.05$, $1 - \beta = 90\%$ then for $\delta = 0.10$, 1020 patients are required. However, for $\delta = 0.05$, 4014 patients are required. This is nearly four times as many! We can also see from this table that a change in $1 - \beta$ from 80% to 90% can also influence n, although in not as marked a manner as changes in δ. Finally, large changes in our estimate of an appropriate π_C can also have a considerable influence on n.

The uncertainty in the specification of the components and their subsequent influence on the calculations, taken together with the necessary assumption of proportional hazards used for the calculations, serves to emphasise that sample size calculations provide no more than a guide to the number of patients that may be required.

ANTICIPATED OR MINIMAL CLINICALLY RELEVANT BENEFIT?

Throughout this chapter we have presented sample size calculations based on an anticipated benefit. Thus, for example, $\delta = \pi_T - \pi_C$ is presented as the difference between test and control that it is anticipated will be observed. An alternative to this is to argue that δ should be set as the 'minimal clinically relevant benefit' or the 'difference worth detecting'. Parmar et al. (1994) give a fuller discussion of these issues.

Example

In the confirmatory trial planned following the results obtained by Valerius *et al.* (1991) we previously considered designing a trial with an anticipated benefit of $\delta = 0.35$. Suppose, however, we consider this may be too optimistic and regard $\delta = 0.20$ as a more realistic anticipated benefit. Thus we replace the anticipated benefit by, in this case, a smaller anticipated benefit, but one which we think is nevertheless of clinical relevance. In doing this we are stating that: 'A benefit at least as large as 0.20 will be of clinical importance'. The effect of replacing $\delta = 0.35$ by $\delta = 0.20$ whilst retaining the same test size and power increases the number of patients required from n = 88 to n = 258.

BALANCING ACCRUAL AND FOLLOW-UP

We have noted earlier that it is the total number of events that determines the power of the study or equivalently the power of the subsequent logrank test. For any study with a survival time endpoint there is clearly a period of accrual during which subjects are recruited to a study and a further period of follow-up beyond the end of accrual during which time more events are observed. To observe a pre-specified number of events we can either (i) keep the accrual period as short as possible and extend follow-up; or (ii) keep the accrual period as long as practicable and have a short post-recruitment follow-up; or (iii) achieve a balance between accrual and follow-up. The approach taken depends on the scarcity of subjects available for study, the event rate in the control arm and practical considerations, such as the costs of accrual and follow-up. For example, in rare diseases it may be considered that it is best to minimise the number of patients required while maximising the follow-up period. Alternatively, in a more common disease it may be more appropriate to minimise the total study time, which comprises the sum of the accrual and follow-up periods, to observe the required number of events.

UNEQUAL ALLOCATION

In the situations presented above we have assumed that equal numbers of patients are to be randomised to each of the two alternative treatments. If, however, the allocation is to be in the ratio of a:b, or $\phi:1$, where $\phi = a/b$, rather than 1:1 in the test and control groups, then the total number of events required to be observed is given by

$$E = [(z_{1-\alpha/2} + z_{1-\beta})(1 + \phi\Delta)/(1 - \Delta)]^2/\phi. \qquad (10.11)$$

The corresponding total number of subjects is

$$n = (1 + \phi)E/[\phi(1 - \pi_T) + (1 - \pi_C)]. \qquad (10.12)$$

Example

Suppose in the confirmatory trial using the anti-pseudomonas therapy in patients with cystic fibrosis the investigators had decided that, since the proposed therapy is new, they may require some experience with the therapy itself whereas they are very familiar with the (no treatment) control therapy. In such a situation it may be appropriate to randomise patients in blocks of five in a ratio of 3:2 in favour of the test treatment, i.e. 3 patients receiving T for every 2 receiving C.

In this case, a = 3, b = 2 and $\phi = 3/2 = 1.5$. Use of equations (10.11) and (10.12) with two-sided $\alpha = 0.05$, $1 - \beta = 0.80$, $\pi_C = 0.50$ and $\pi_T = 0.85$ gives a total of n = 67 or 70 patients to the nearest larger integer divisible by the block size of five. Thus dividing these in a ratio of 3:2 gives 42 to receive the new treatment and 28 the control. The total of 67 patients is larger than the 62 we had calculated earlier for a 1:1 randomisation.

In general, unless the allocation ratio is more extreme than 2:1, i.e. the value of ϕ is greater than 2, then unequal allocation does not make a substantial difference to the number of events and subjects required.

LOSS TO FOLLOW-UP

One aspect of a trial which can affect the number of patients recruited is the proportion of patients who are subsequently lost to follow-up during the trial. Since these patients are lost, we will never observe and record the date of the critical event, even though it may have occurred. Such patients have censored observations, in the same way as those for whom the event of interest has still not occurred by the time of analysis of the trial. Such lost patients do not, and will never, contribute events for the analysis and, therefore, we need to compensate for their loss. If the anticipated loss or withdrawal rate is x or 100x%, then the required number of patients, n, given by either equations (10.10) or (10.12) should be increased to

$$n_{Adjusted} = n/(1 - x). \tag{10.13}$$

Example

An adjuvant study of the drug levamisole is proposed for patients with resectable cancer of the colon (Dukes' C), in which the primary objective of the study is to compare the efficacy of levamisole against a placebo control, with respect to relapse-free survival. How many patients need to be recruited in the trial if a decrease from 50% to 40% in relapse rates at 1 year is anticipated, and a power of 80% is required? A patient loss rate of 10% is anticipated.

Here we wish to increase the success rate, i.e. failure to relapse, from 50% to 60%, so $\pi_C = 0.5$ and $\pi_T = 0.6$. These give $\delta = 0.6 - 0.5 = 0.1$ and $\Delta = \log 0.6/\log 0.5 = 0.74$. Assuming a two-sided test with $\alpha = 0.05$, $1 - \beta = 0.8$, and equal randomisation $\phi = 1$, then Table T4, with $\pi_C = 0.5$ and $\delta = 0.1$, gives n = 764 patients required.

Allowing for a loss to follow-up rate x = 10% and using equation (10.13) we obtain $n_{Adjusted} = 849$. Thus, a total of approximately 850 subjects should be recruited to the trial, half of whom will receive levamisole.

10.6 THE POWER OF A GIVEN STUDY

In certain circumstances, it may not be possible to recruit as many subjects to a study as the ideal design demands. In this case, it may be sensible to ask: with the n patients available what chance is there of detecting the anticipated benefit? This can be alternatively expressed as; what is the power of the proposed study?

The power can be obtained for given π_C, π_T, n and α by combining equations (10.11) and (10.12) into one expression to give

$$z_{1-\beta} = \frac{(1-\Delta)\sqrt{\{n\phi[\phi(1-\pi_T) + (1-\pi_C)]/(1+\phi)\}}}{(1+\phi\Delta)} - z_{1-\alpha/2}. \tag{10.14}$$

Example

Assuming a two-sided comparison with $\alpha = 0.05$, what is the power of the trial conducted by Valerius et al. (1991)?

For their trial $n = 26$, $n_C = 12$, $n_T = 14$ and so $\phi = 14/12 = 1.17$. Their results also suggest $\pi_T = 0.85$ and $\pi_C = 0.5$ and hence $\Delta = \log 0.85/\log 0.50 = 0.23$. Finally, with $\alpha = 0.05$ we have from Table T2 that $z_{0.975} = 1.96$.

Thus, from equation (10.13) we have

$$z_{1-\beta} = \frac{(1-0.23)\sqrt{\{26 \times 1.17[1.17(1-0.85) + (1-0.5)]/2.17\}}}{(1+1.17 \times 0.23)} - 1.96$$

$$= 1.6246 - 1.96 = -0.3354 \approx -0.34$$

Referring to Table T1, this corresponds to an area of 0.7339 in the two tails of the Normal distribution or $0.7339/2 = 0.3670$ in each tail. As a consequence, the power, which is the area below $z = -0.3354$, is $1 - \beta = 1 - 0.3670 = 0.63$ or 63%. This suggests that such a trial would only have approximately a two in three (~66%) chance of detecting a difference as large as the postulated $\delta = 0.35$ or $\Delta = 0.23$. In normal circumstances we would not embark on a trial with such a lack of power.

10.7   CALCULATIONS ASSUMING EXPONENTIAL SURVIVAL

If we can assume that survival times in the two groups are exponentially distributed, rather than have just proportional hazards, then the number of events required to give a test size α and power $1 - \beta$ is, for an equally allocated two-group trial

$$E = [(z_{1-\alpha/2} + z_{1-\beta})(2/\log \Delta)]^2. \tag{10.15}$$

This can be contrasted with equation (10.8). Note that the assumption of exponential survival distributions, which implies constant hazards within each of the two groups, is a more restrictive assumption than that of proportional hazards. The assumption of constant hazards is, of course, a special case of the assumption of proportional hazards. Collett (1994, p. 265) has pointed out that for small values of log Δ equations (10.8) and (10.15) will be approximately equivalent because

$$2/(\log \Delta) \simeq (1 + \Delta)/(1 - \Delta). \tag{10.16}$$

Thus, for small log Δ, i.e. for small to moderate effect sizes, the proportional hazards assumption and the exponential survival distributions assumption will produce similar study sizes. For this reason, and the rather less restrictive assumption of proportional hazards, we recommend the use of equation (10.8) and hence Table T4 for the sample size.

11 Miscellaneous Topics

Summary

Several topics are introduced in which standard methods of survival analysis have been adapted to allow different analyses to be performed. These include the analysis of contraceptive follow-up studies where there are usually a number of endpoints of interest. These endpoints are often given equal emphasis when interpreting the results of such studies.

An example of the analysis of paired survival data is presented in the context of analysing data from a crossover trial. The methods of meta-analysis—the approach of combining the results from similar trials—as applied survival data, are briefly presented. Application of regression analysis techniques to the (parametric) exponential and Weibull models are described and a comparison is made with the (non-parametric) Cox model. Finally, the use of survival methods in sequential trials are briefly described.

11.1 CONTRACEPTIVE STUDIES

Clinical trials of contraceptive methods are a major area in which survival methods have been used and adapted. The primary objective of a contraceptive method is to permit intercourse but prevent conception, thereby allowing planned parenthood. A failure of a contraceptive method is an unplanned pregnancy whilst using the method. However, current studies of contraceptive efficacy and use effectiveness differ from other medical areas in that there is often no single primary endpoint.

Typically, subjects in a contraceptive study are healthy women aged between 20 and 45 years and the incidence of pregnancy among such women is high in the absence of any contraceptive method. However, the efficacy of contraceptive drugs or devices under trial is also very high. Thus annual pregnancy rates among intrauterine device (IUD) users range from 2–10%, whereas the corresponding rates among women not using contraceptives, and who are exposed to the risk of pregnancy, are 80–90%. One consequence of such low pregnancy rates is that any randomised trials, comparing contraceptive methods using conception as the sole endpoint (event) of interest, will have to be very large in order that the required number of events is observed. As a result it is usual to define additional endpoints in these trials. We return to this point when discussing the data of Table 11.1 below.

The method of protection against pregnancy may be interrupted for a number of reasons. For an IUD, for example, the most common reasons may be the involuntary expulsion of the device or its removal following a complaint of uterine pain and/or bleeding. Although these, and other endpoints indicating lack of satisfaction with the method, may be considered side-effects, they are an essential feature in the assessment of the efficacy of the device. For example, an IUD which gives excellent protection against pregnancy but has a high expulsion rate may not be as attractive as a device which remains *in situ* but gives a lower protection against pregnancy.

Until relatively recently, data from contraceptive studies have been analysed in grouped time intervals corresponding to the scheduled follow-up patterns described in the trial protocol. This was because certain endpoints, for example conception, may not be dated exactly. As a consequence, the approximate timing of these events encouraged the use of the actuarial or grouped time method of analysis described in section 2.13. However, current practice is to date the events as precisely as possible and to use continuous time for analysis.

THE PEARL RATE

In a contraceptive study, one main focus is overall protection against pregnancy. Thus, subjects who are contraceptive failures, i.e. they conceive, are the subjects who experience 'events' in the study. The first reports on contraceptive effectiveness used the Pearl rate (PR) to summarise pregnancy rates. This is defined as

$$PR = \frac{\text{Number of pregnancies observed (conceptions)}}{\text{Total method experience (years)}}. \qquad (11.1)$$

It is often multiplied by 100 and expressed as per 100 years of exposure or method use. Equation (11.1) corresponds exactly to equation (3.4), which was used to estimate the constant hazard of the exponential distribution, since the total method experience will consist of the sum of both censored and non-censored times to conception. The advantage of such an index is that it is very easily calculated and also readily understood. However, the assumption of a constant pregnancy rate with time is not generally true for contraceptive users. For example, it is biologically established that the risk of pregnancy shortly after childbirth is very small. A further problem is that subjects of high fertility will become pregnant soon after the start of their period on the trial and so the observed pregnancy rate relative to the day 0 of randomisation to a trial is likely to decline as this 'high risk' group is removed from the study population.

Thus, although frequently used, the PR is not often a relevant statistic for contraceptive studies. It can sometimes be appropriate for very rare events, such as ectopic pregnancies, for which there are insufficient data to detect departures from the assumption of a constant risk. Additionally, since it was the standard measure for many years, continued use of the PR provides a link to earlier studies.

Example from the literature

The World Health Organization Task Force for the Regulation of Male Fertility (1990) report one pregnancy arising from 1486 months of exposure to pregnancy in partners of men who were receiving injections to induce azoospermia so as to render them effectively infertile. They calculated, therefore, $PR = [1/(1486/12)] \times 100 = 1200/1486 = 0.8075$ pregnancies per 100 years of exposure.

In addition to the principal endpoint of pregnancy in the female partner, several secondary endpoints were also recorded. These secondary endpoints were essentially the reasons given by the men for not receiving the next scheduled injection. Such endpoints are often described as discontinuation reasons. The PR corresponding to the six different reasons for method discontinuation including pregnancy are summarised in Table 11.1.

In each of the distinct calculations, only the subjects experiencing the event of interest, say injection difficulties, have uncensored survival times. Those discontinuing the method for other reasons, including pregnancy, have censored survival times with respect to this particular event. In addition, it is quite common to calculate the PR for 'all discontinuations' as an overall measure of the discontinuation rate of the method under study. The corresponding $PR = 30.7$ for the 38 events.

To calculate a confidence interval (CI) for a PR we can use equation (3.7) with equation (3.9), provided the number of events, d, is relatively large. It is clear,

Table 11.1   Pearl rates for conception and other reasons for discontinuation in a study to investigate the acceptability of injections to induce azoospermia (infertility) in the male partner (From World Health Organization Task Force for the Regulation of Male Fertility, 1990, Contraceptive efficacy of testosterone-induced azoospermia in normal men. *Lancet* 336, 955–959, © by The Lancet Ltd)

Reason for method discontinuation	Number of events	Pearl rate (PR)	95% CI
Pregnancy	1	0.8	0.0–4.5
Injection difficulties	7	5.7	2.3–11.6
Medical reasons	14	11.3	6.2–19.0
Personal reasons	13	10.5	5.6–17.9
Protocol violation	2	1.6	0.2–5.8
Loss to follow-up	1	0.8	0.0–4.5
All discontinuations	38	30.7	21.7–42.1

however, for the one pregnancy of Table 11.1 that numbers are not large. In such a situation, the so-called exact CIs have to be calculated. These can be obtained from statistical tables such as those of Geigy Scientific Tables, Volume 2 (Lenter, 1991, p. 152). The 95% CI of 0.0 to 4.5 per 100 years of IUD use, quoted in Table 11.1, was obtained from these tables.

If we use equations (3.7) and (3.9) to obtain a 95% CI for the PR corresponding to, for example, the 14 discontinuations for medical reasons then we obtain 5.2 to 17.4 per 100 years of IUD use. In this case there are a relatively large number of events and the CI is quite close to the exact CI of 6.2 to 19.0 given in Table 11.1. If there is any doubt as to whether to use equations (3.7) and (3.9) or exact statistical tables to calculate CIs, then the latter are to be preferred.

The PR has also been used in studies comparing two methods of contraception. In this situation the PR is calculated for each method on trial and a statistical test of the null hypothesis of no difference in PRs is made.

Example from the literature

In a report from the Oxford Family Planning Association Contraceptive Study by Vessey *et al.* (1976), covering the period from May 1968 to April 1975, the PR was used as the measure of contraceptive use effectiveness. They report on two types of the Lippes Loop IUD (A or B versus C or D) and their results are summarised in Table 11.2. We refer to these groups as LL1 and LL2 IUDs.

The null hypothesis of equal PRs is tested by assuming that the total number of pregnancies observed, C, can be attributed to one of the two types of IUD according to the degree of exposure in each group. In this approach we first calculate the overall pregnancy (Pearl) rate as $PR_{Overall} = (C/Y) \times 100$, and then apply this rate to the exposure in groups LL1 and LL2, respectively. This gives the expected number of pregnancies as $E_1 = Y_1 \times (C/Y)$ and $E_2 = Y_2 \times (C/Y)$.

This method is analogous to the way we apportion each successive observed death, in Table 4.4, into the expected deaths attributable to the two treatments, A and B, when calculating the logrank test of equation (4.3). The difference here is that the denominator is the total number of years of IUD use in the particular group, rather than the number of subjects at risk at time, t, in that group.

Table 11.2 Use effectiveness of IUDs investigated in the Oxford Family Planning Association Study (From Vessey *et al.*, 1976. Reproduced by permission of *Journal of Biosocial Science*)

	Lippes Loop IUD		
	A or B (LL1)	C or D (LL2)	Total
Number of pregnancies	17 (C_1)	101 (C_2)	118 (C)
Woman years of observation	416 (Y_1)	5249 (Y_2)	5665 (Y)
PR	4.087	1.924	2.083

The observed and expected values can then be compared in the usual χ^2 test of equations (1.14) or (4.3), with $df = 1$ since there are $g = 2$ groups. Thus

$$\chi^2 = \frac{(C_1 - E_1)^2}{E_1} + \frac{(C_2 - E_2)^2}{E_2}. \tag{11.2}$$

Example

To test whether the PR associated with the two types of IUD of Table 11.2 differs, we calculate $PR_{Overall} = (118/5665) \times 100 = 2.0830$, $E_1 = 416 \times 0.020830 = 8.6653$ and $E_2 = 5249 \times 0.020830 = 109.3367$. Finally, substituting these values together with $C_1 = 17$ and $C_2 = 101$ in equation (11.2) gives $\chi^2 = 8.6644$.

Use of Table T3, with $df = 1$, suggests a p-value <0.01. More exact calculation, from Table T1, with $z = \sqrt{8.6644} = 2.94$, gives a p-value $= 0.002$. This result suggests there is a statistically significant difference with a lower PR for those using the Lippes Loop IUDs C or D.

HAZARD RATIO

As we have indicated in earlier chapters the ratio of two relative hazards estimates the HR. Thus, in this context, this can be estimated by the ratio of two PRs, or

$$HR = PR_2/PR_1. \tag{11.3}$$

Example

The PR for the LL2 IUDs of Table 11.2 is approximately half that observed for those of LL1 since $HR = 1.924/4.087 = 0.4708$.

A CI for the HR, estimated from the ratio of two PRs, is given by

$$\exp[(1 + z_{1-\alpha/2}/\sqrt{\chi^2})\log HR] \quad \text{to} \quad \exp[(1 - z_{1-\alpha/2}/\sqrt{\chi^2})\log HR], \tag{11.4}$$

where $z_{1-\alpha/2}$ is the percentile of the standard Normal distribution.

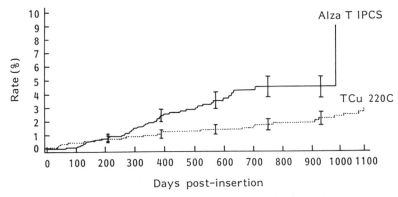

Figure 11.1 Cumulative pregnancy rate by IUD type using the Kaplan–Meier or daily life table method (From Farley, 1986, with permission)

We note in equation (11.4) that the expressions for the lower and upper values of the CI differ only in the sign that follows 1. In this case, and in contrast to equation (2.9) for example, the +sign appears within the left-hand expression and the −sign in the right.

This CI is called a test-based CI as it uses the value of the computed test statistic χ^2 of equation (11.2) in the calculation.

Example

Using the data from Table 11.2, we have $HR = 1.924/4.087 = 0.4708$. The 95% CI for the HR, from equation (11.4) and using $\chi^2 = 8.6644$, is obtained from the use of equation (11.2):

$$\exp\{(1 + 1.96/\sqrt{8.6644})\log 0.4708\} \quad \text{to} \quad \exp\{(1 - 1.96/\sqrt{8.6644})\log 0.4708\}$$

or

$$\exp\{(1 + 0.6659) \times (-0.7533)\} \quad \text{to} \quad \exp\{(1 - 0.6659) \times (-0.7533)\}$$

and finally

$$\exp(-1.2549) = 0.29 \quad \text{to} \quad \exp(-0.2517) = 0.78.$$

This 95% CI suggests rather convincing evidence of the better use effectiveness of the LL2 IUDs since the upper end of the confidence interval is distant from the null hypothesis value, $HR = 1$.

CUMULATIVE PREGNANCY RATE

Kaplan–Meier or daily life table estimates can be used in contraceptive studies with pregnancy as an outcome. However, it is usual to present these in a cumulative pregnancy rate format, which in fact is just [1 − (Kaplan–Meier estimate)].

Example from the literature

The statistical methods appropriate to contraceptive research are discussed by Farley (1986), who applied the Kaplan–Meier method to data from a large study on 2514 women comparing two IUDs. These were a standard reference device, TCu 220c, and a new experimental steroid-releasing device, the Alza T IPCS 52. The cumulative pregnancy rates are shown in Figure 11.1. The estimate of the cumulative pregnancy rate at 2 years is approximately 4% with Alza T IPCS 52, but only 1.5% with TCu 220c.

Farley (1986) compared these Kaplan–Meier calculations with parallel ones using grouped data (see section 2.13) which had often been used in contraceptive development studies. He showed that the conclusions drawn were materially the same and that this would often be the case with the two approaches.

However, the continuous time (more strictly daily) Kaplan–Meier approach summarised in Figure 11.1 also permits the use of Cox proportional hazards models to investigate the possible influence of variables, such as the characteristics of the subjects themselves, on discontinuation rates.

The calculations of the associated HR, logrank test and CIs are given by the methods described in chapter 4. The only difference for a contraceptive study is that these are usually constructed for each discontinuation reason or group of discontinuation reasons separately.

DISCONTINUATION REASONS

An example of the types of discontinuation reasons that are appropriate to an injectable contraceptive for the male have been indicated in Table 11.1. The types of event usually considered as endpoints for an IUD study are listed in Table 11.3. There are two broad categories: one of use-related discontinuations, and the second of other discontinuations. The 'use-related' discontinuations are regarded as pertaining to measures of the efficacy of the device and are usually reported both separately and combined.

The remaining discontinuation reasons are features that are included in measures of overall performance or use effectiveness. Although these categories of discontinuation are mutually exclusive they do not necessarily represent independent risks. It is essential to consider the discontinuation reasons both individually and also by grouping into related categories, when interpreting contraceptive data.

It is common practice to quote cumulative discontinuation rates, for each discontinuation reason, separately and for all reasons combined (as in Table 11.1, in which PRs were presented).

Example from the literature

Table 11.4 shows the 12-month cumulative discontinuation rates, for 10 distinct

Table 11.3 Types of event leading to discontinuation of the method for IUD trials (From Farley, 1986, with permission)

Use-related discontinuations
   Pregnancy
      Intrauterine
      Extrauterine
   Expulsion
   Perforation
   Medical removals
      Pain alone
      Bleeding alone
      Pain and bleeding
      Pelvic inflammatory disease
      Other
Non-medical removals
   Wish to become pregnant
   No further need
   Other
Loss to follow-up
Other reasons

Table 11.4 Twelve-month cumulative discontinuation rates (%) in women using 100 or 150 mg DMPA in four 3-monthly injections (after WHO Task Force on Long-acting Systemic Agents for Fertility Regulation, 1986)

Discontinuation reason	DMPA (mg)	
	100	150
Unwanted pregnancy	0.4	0.0
Amenorrhoea	7.2	12.5
Prolonged bleeding	7.7	7.7
Irregular bleeding	3.3	3.1
Heavy bleeding	3.4	1.2
Spotting	1.1	1.8
Other medical reasons	5.1	4.3
Desires pregnancy	2.5	1.3
Other non-medical reasons	11.1	9.9
Lost to follow-up	8.2	8.6
All reasons	40.7	41.2
Number of women	609	607

discontinuation reasons, in 1216 female users of depot-medroxyprogesterone acetate (DMPA) randomised to receive four 3-monthly injections at a dose of either 100 or 150 mg (WHO Task Force on Long-acting Systemic Agents for Fertility Regulation, 1986).

It is clear from Table 11.4 that the unwanted cumulative pregnancy rates are similar and very small with each dose (0.4% and 0.0%). However, the overall or 'all reasons' discontinuation rates are high, although very similar, at 41%. Nevertheless, there are different patterns for some discontinuation reasons with, for example, an indication of increased discontinuation for amenorrhoea with the 150 mg injection.

It should be noted that 'lost to follow-up' is regarded as an event. This is because, in contraceptive trials, one method of expressing dissatisfaction with a method is not to return for the next follow-up visit, at which time it had been planned to supply the contraceptive for the following period of the study. For example, the clinic may intend to distribute oral contraceptive (OC) supplies for the next few months once the woman had been given a routine medical examination following a period of OC use.

Thus, in many contraceptive studies, the only truly censored observations arise from subjects who complete the study without discontinuing method use. In these women no 'events' have occurred in any of the categories of Table 11.4. It is common for contraceptive efficacy trials to have a fixed duration. Thus the trial we have just described recruited women to receive a maximum of four injections providing contraceptive cover for 1 year and follow-up ceases at this anniversary. On completion of the year those women who had not discontinued the method earlier provide the only truly censored observations.

TIME TO EVENT

It is important to determine the time to the critical event as precisely as possible. As is customary in other situations, the date of randomisation defines day 0 but the event date may not always be so easily identified. Thus although the exact number of days between insertion and discontinuation can be determined easily in cases of removal of an IUD, conventions are required for pregnancies, expulsions and perforations.

The number of days to pregnancy is either computed from the date at which the subject thought she was pregnant, the date of confirmation of pregnancy or the estimated date of conception. Expulsions can either be complete, in that the device is expelled entirely from the uterus, or partial, in that it is only dislodged from the correct position. In both cases, the day the expulsion was noticed is usually used. Perforations are treated in a similar way. If a pregnancy occurs with a complete or partial expulsion then this is regarded as a pregnancy; if a large number of such events occurs a special class of 'pregnancy with expulsion' is made. For those lost to follow-up, the time of the last contact with the subject is usually taken as the discontinuation date.

Categories of reasons for discontinuation, generally considered in injectable contraceptive studies in women, present an additional problem since contraceptive efficacy lasts for a considerable number of days (often 90) following the injection. Pregnancies within this period are very rare and those accidental pregnancies that do occur usually do so when a subject is late for her repeat injection. Moreover, many of the women who discontinue the method may not in fact return to the clinic. As a consequence, reasons for not wanting a further injection cannot be ascertained. Since the efficacy of the method continues for 90 days it is reasonable to regard such a woman as lost to follow-up from the time of the first missed follow-up visit or 90 days from the last injection, whichever is the shorter.

Example from the literature

Figure 11.2 shows the cumulative discontinuation rate for 'all reasons' in the trial conducted by the WHO Task Force on Long-acting Systemic Agents for Fertility Regulation (1986), which compares 3-monthly DMPA, at doses of 100 and 150 mg, in 1216 women.

As noted earlier, injections are given four times in the study period of 1 year. Once an injection is given, the woman has 3 months' protection. The Kaplan–Meier estimate of the cumulative rates clearly illustrates the 3-month plateau between successive steps. The fact that the steps are not precisely rectangular reflects the reality of follow-up visits, which may not be exactly at 3 months. For example, clinic visits may be every 4 weeks, so for practical purposes 3 months is, in many cases, 12 weeks rather than 13. A second reason is that any pregnancies will be assigned an estimated conception date which may be at any time in the 3-month interval. The all reasons discontinuation rate is approximately 40% at 1 year for both methods, as we noted earlier.

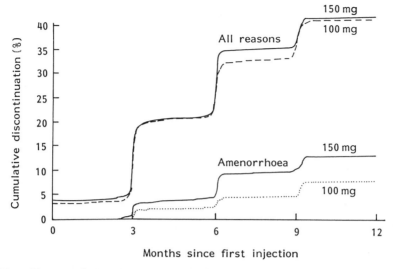

Figure 11.2 The cumulative discontinuation rates for all reasons, including women lost to follow-up (upper curves) and for amenorrhoea (lower curves), by dose of DMPA (from World Health Organization Task Force on Long-acting Systemic Agents for Fertility Regulation, 1986)

In this trial there was a particular interest in discontinuations for amenorrhoea and this is why the corresponding cumulative discontinuation rates for the two methods were included in Figure 11.2. As we have already indicated, there is some evidence (see also Table 11.4) of more discontinuations for this reason in the higher dose group.

11.2 PAIRED OBSERVATIONS

As we have indicated previously, survival methods have been developed principally from the study of mortality, particularly cancer mortality, in human populations. Clinical trials to investigate the effect of interventions on such endpoints are generally designed as parallel group studies, in which two or more groups are compared with regard to endpoints such as disease recurrence or death. In these situations, because of the nature of the disease many and usually all patients, will not return to a condition similar to that observed at the time of randomisation. Clearly, in such circumstances, a two-period crossover trial in which patients, for example, receive both therapies under test, either in the order A followed by B, or B followed by A, is not usually appropriate. This is because it is assumed in such designs that once the first treatment is completed patients return to baseline values following an interval in which neither treatment is given (a washout period). Such a return to baseline is very unlikely in patients receiving therapy for a life-threatening disease such as cancer. However, in certain circumstances crossover trials including 'survival' time endpoints may be appropriate. Readers are referred to the book by Senn (1993), which reviews many aspects of crossover trial methodology in a medical context.

Example from the literature

Gross and Lam (1981) describe the analysis of a study for the relief of headaches in which 10 patients received either the standard (S) or new treatment (N) in two successive attacks. The patients record the time to achieve relief with both therapies and the results are summarised in Table 11.5.

Although Gross and Lam (1981) do not give details, the standard and new treatments for headache relief may have been given to five patients, chosen at random from the 10, in the order SN and to the remainder in the order NS. There is an assumption here that the intervals between successive headaches are such that the effect of the particular drug given during the first episode will no longer be present during the second. We note, from Table 11.5, that the times to headache relief with N tend to be shorter, i.e. bring quicker relief to the patient, than with S. Since all patients obtained headache relief there are no censored headache times.

Example from the literature

France *et al.* (1991) describe a crossover trial to compare the efficacy of atenolol (A) alone, with that of a combination of atenolol and nifedipine (C), in patients with angina pectoris. The trial design is summarised in Figure 11.3. Briefly, all patients underwent a run-in period on atenolol alone of 4 weeks. Patients then underwent an exercise test and were selected for entry into the randomised component of the study. Randomisation was to 4 weeks of A followed by 4 weeks of C, or 4 weeks of C followed by 4 weeks of A. There was no 'washout' period. That is, there was no delay before switching to the other treatment because neither treatment was

Table 11.5 Times to relief of headaches for standard (S) and new (N) treatments (min) (From Gross and Lam, 1981, with permission.)

Patients	Treatment		Difference S – N	Preference
	Standard S	New N		
1	8.4	6.9	1.5	N
2	7.7	6.8	0.9	N
3	10.1	10.3	−0.2	S
4	9.6	9.4	0.2	N
5	9.3	8.0	1.3	N
6	9.1	8.8	0.3	N
7	9.0	6.1	2.9	N
8	7.7	7.4	0.3	N
9	8.1	8.0	0.1	N
10	5.3	5.1	0.2	N

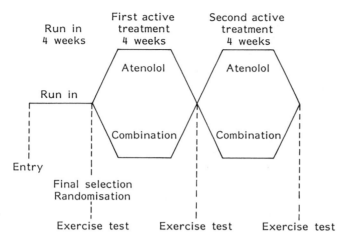

Figure 11.3 Design of a two-period crossover trial of atenolol and the combination atenolol plus nifedipine, for patients with angina pectoris (reproduced from France *et al.*, 1991, with permission)

expected to have a carryover effect which persisted beyond the end of the 4 week treatment period. At the end of each treatment period the patients performed a treadmill exercise test, in which the patient's ECG (electrocardiogram) was monitored. Using this, the time to 1 mm ST segment depression was recorded for each patient. Patients stopped the test when they suffered excessive anginal pain, tiredness, breathlessness or other symptoms, and thus generated censored times for attaining 1 mm ST segment depression.

We note that the survival data we have now is paired because we have two survival times for each subject. One simple method of analysis is to count patient 'preferences'. Thus patients who experience an event on one treatment in a shorter time than they experience it on the other are said to 'prefer' that treatment. However, there are three situations in which a patient preference cannot be determined. Two of these arise from censored observations being present. In the first situation the event of interest may not occur before the observation period is complete on either treatment. In the second, the event may occur on one treatment only, but this event time occurs after the time at which observation was stopped on the other treatment for a different reason. These situations are described as providing 'no information'. The third situation is when there is a tie, in that the event occurs with the same survival time with each treatment. In this case there is 'no preference'.

If we can assume that the survival times in the two treatments of a crossover trial give proportional hazards then France *et al.* (1991) estimate the HR by

$$\text{HR} = \frac{\text{Number of preferences for treatment 1}}{\text{Number of preferences for treatment 2}}. \tag{11.5}$$

With this estimate we assume that period effects can be ignored. That is, the effect of treatment 1 is the same whether it precedes or follows treatment 2. This similarly applies for treatment 2 preceded or followed by treatment 1.

Example from the literature

In the example of Gross and Lam (1981) summarised in Table 11.5, there are no tied or censored observations. There were nine patients who preferred the new therapy and one the standard. As a consequences the HR for assessing S against N for the relief of headache can be estimated from equation (11.5) as HR = 9/1 = 9.0.

Example from the literature

The preferences recorded in the trial in patients with angina pectoris and described by France et al. (1991) are summarised in Table 11.6.

Of the 106 patients completing the trial there are three patients who provide no preference and 15 who provide no information. Ignoring these 18 cases gives, from equation (11.5), an estimate of the HR = 62/26 = 2.385 in favour of the combination therapy C.

COX MODEL

A trial such as that described by France et al. (1991) is called a two-period, two-treatment, crossover trial. Such a trial can be summarised by use of the Cox proportional hazards regression model, in which each patient has a separate underlying hazard which is influenced by both treatment (A or B) and period (I or II). Thus, we can specify the relative hazard as

$$h = \exp(\beta_T x_T + \beta_P x_P).\tag{11.6}$$

Here $x_T = 0$ for treatment A, and $x_T = 1$ for treatment B, while $x_P = 0$ for period I and $x_P = 1$ for period II. Note, that this is of the same form as equation (6.18). The regression coefficients β_T and β_P correspond to the treatment and period effects, respectively. Thus $HR_T = \exp(\beta_T)$ and $HR_P = \exp(\beta_P)$.

We assume n_{AB} patients are randomised to receive the sequence AB and n_{BA} to receive the sequence BA, giving a total of $n_{AB} + n_{BA}$ patients recruited to the crossover trial. Further, amongst the n_{AB} patients there are $n_{AB,A}$ who prefer A and

Table 11.6   Patient preferences for atenolol or the combination obtained by comparing paired treadmill exercise times in patients with angina pectoris (reproduced from France et al., 1991 with permission)

Preference	Number of patients
Combination (C)	62
Atenolol (A)	26
No preference	3
No information	15
Total	106

$n_{AB,B}$ who prefer B. Similarly, there are amongst the n_{BA} patients $n_{BA,A}$ who prefer A and $n_{BA,B}$ who prefer B. Using this notation it can be shown that maximum likelihood estimates of the HRs are

$$HR_T = \sqrt{\left(\frac{n_{AB,B}n_{BA,B}}{n_{AB,A}n_{BA,A}}\right)}$$

(11.7)

and

$$HR_P = \sqrt{\left(\frac{n_{AB,A}n_{BA,B}}{n_{AB,B}n_{BA,A}}\right)}.$$

(11.8)

Details of expressions for the corresponding SEs are given by France *et al.* (1991).

Example from the literature

In the crossover trial described by France *et al.* (1991) $n_{AC} = 54$ patients completed the sequence AC. Of these $n_{AC,A} = 12$ preferred A, and $n_{AC,C} = 33$ preferred C, with nine patients providing ties or no information. Similarly $n_{CA} = 52$ patients completed the sequence CA, of which $n_{CA,A} = 14$ preferred A, and $n_{CA,C} = 29$ preferred C, again with nine providing ties or no information. Substituting these values in equations (11.7) and (11.8) respectively gives

$$HR_T = \sqrt{\left(\frac{33}{12} \times \frac{29}{14}\right)} = 2.387$$

and

$$HR_P = \sqrt{\left(\frac{12}{33} \times \frac{29}{14}\right)} = 0.868.$$

The estimate $HR_T = 2.387$ is very similar to the estimate $HR = 2.385$, obtained by using equation (11.5), which took no account of any difference between periods. This small difference in the two estimates reflects the lack of a period effect in these data. This is further emphasised by $HR_P = 0.868$, which is close to the null hypothesis value presenting no period effect or $HR_P = 1$.

SURVIVAL CURVES

In a crossover trial, or in other circumstances that may provide paired survival data, the Kaplan–Meier estimates of the survival curves for each treatment can be calculated in the usual way. However, in such a calculation every patient contributes to both curves but no account is taken of the paired nature of the data. These curves, therefore, do not make the best use of the information available. This is analogous to using a two-sample t-test, rather than a paired t-test when the design indicates the latter should be used.

To overcome this difficulty France *et al.* (1991) suggest that survival curves for all observations on each treatment A and B are calculated separately and are then combined into an average survivor function $S_{Average}(t)$. The average is calculated from

$$S_{Average}(t) = \sqrt{[S_A(t)S_B(t)]} \tag{11.9}$$

where $S_A(t)$ and $S_B(t)$ are the Kaplan–Meier estimates for all observations on treatments A and B, respectively. Using this average survival curve, the individual survival curves for each treatment group are then calculated as

$$S_A^*(t) = [S_{Average}(t)]^{\exp(+\beta_T/2)}$$

and   (11.10)

$$S_B^*(t) = [S_{Average}(t)]^{\exp(-\beta_T/2)}$$

where β_T is as defined in equation (11.6).

Example

To illustrate this procedure we use the data on the relief of headaches summarised in Table 11.5. The data are repeated in Table 11.7 but in an ordered format similar to that used to calculate both the Kaplan–Meier curves (Table 2.2) and the logrank test (Table 4.3).

Table 11.7 Calculation of the survival curves corresponding to two successive treatments given to 10 patients for the relief of headache (From Gross and Lam, 1981, with permission.)

Standard		New				
t (min)	$S_S(t)$	t (min)	$S_N(t)$	$S_{Average}(t)$	$S_S^*(t)$	$S_N^*(t)$
0	1	0	1	1	1	1
	[1]	5.1	0.9	0.9487	0.9826	0.8539
5.3	0.9		[0.9]	0.9000	0.9655	0.7290
	[0.9]	6.1	0.8	0.8485	0.9467	0.6109
	[0.9]	6.8	0.7	0.7397	0.9259	0.5000
	[0.9]	6.9	0.6	0.7348	0.9024	0.3967
	[0.9]	7.4	0.5	0.6708	0.8754	0.3018
7.7,7.7	0.7		[0.5]	0.5916	0.8395	0.2071
	[0.7]	8.0,8.0	0.3	0.4583	0.7710	0.0963
8.1	0.6		[0.3]	0.4243	0.7514	0.0764
8.4	0.5		[0.3]	0.3873	0.7289	0.0581
	[0.5]	8.8	0.2	0.3162	0.6813	0.0316
9.0	0.4		[0.2]	0.2828	0.6564	0.0226
9.1	0.3		[0.2]	0.2449	0.6256	0.0147
9.3	0.2		[0.2]	0.2000	0.5848	0.0080
	[0.2]	9.4	0.1	0.1414	0.5210	0.0028
9.6	0.1		[0.1]	0.1000	0.4642	0.0010
10.1	0.0		[0.1]	0.0000	0.0000	0.0000
	[0.0]	10.3	0.0	0.0000	0.0000	0.0000

In this example there are 10 patients and no censored observations, so that the survival curve estimate at any one time for each treatment is the simple proportion remaining alive at that point. At the times when no events are observed in one treatment but an event is observed with the other, the Kaplan–Meier estimate does not change in the former but decreases in the latter. For example, at $t = 9.0$ min the Kaplan–Meier estimate in treatment S is 0.4 and that with N is 0.2, although the event corresponding to the latter value occurred earlier at time 8.8 min. For clarity we have indicated the such probabilities within square brackets so that there is an estimate indicated at each event time. The average survival function at any time t is the square root of the product $S_S(t)$ and $S_N(t)$, i.e. of columns 2 and 4 of Table 11.7.

We observed earlier that the HR = 9.0 for these data, so $b = \log HR = 2.1792$. From this $\exp(-2.1792/2) = 0.3333 = 1/3$ and $\exp(2.1792/2) = 3$. Thus $S_S^*(t) = [S_{Average}(t)]^{1/3}$ and $S_N^*(t) = [S_{Average}(t)]^3$ are the estimates of the survival curves for treatments S and N, respectively. These columns indicate quite clearly that the patients experience headache relief more quickly with drug N. The median time to relief is 6.8 min with N and approximately 9.5 min with S.

Example from the literature

The resulting estimated survival curves for the patients in the trial described by France et al. (1991) following the methodology they propose are summarised in Figure 11.4. The median exercise time is approximately 300 s with A and 420 s with C. This indicates an increased exercise time by use of the combination therapy.

As we have indicated, a crossover trial is one example which provides paired data and which arises frequently in medicine. Paired, or more accurately matched-pairs, data can be seen in epidemiological follow-up studies. However, pairs also arise naturally in some organs such as eyes, kidneys and ears and their survival either as expressed by loss of sight, kidney dysfunction or loss of hearing, respectively, would generate paired survival times.

Example from the literature

Whitehead and Dorse (1988) describe the Seattle Wolfe Study in which women were screened by mammography for the presence of solid deposits of calcium in the breast. In this study, data were recorded separately for each breast. These women were then followed prospectively for the development of breast cancer in each breast to establish the risk associated with the presence or absence of calcifications in that breast as detected at admission to the study.

In their analysis, they propose a model which includes two hazards: one for 'left disease' and one for 'right disease'. This model then enabled a test of whether any risk due to the presence of calcification was specific to the breast in which the calcification occurs.

A general extension of survival methods from paired organs, such as the kidneys, to consider the time to development of, for example, rheumatoid arthritis in the digits of one hand, both hands or the whole body is clearly possible.

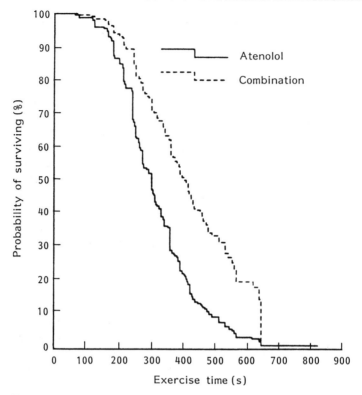

Figure 11.4 Estimated survival curves for 1 mm segment depression based on average survival function and Cox model regression coefficient (From France *et al.*, 1991, with permission.)

Similarly we may consider the time from birth to develop dental caries in each tooth of children.

Example from the literature

Eriksson and Adell (1994) describe a study of stable prosthesis-supporting fixtures with respect to the upper and lower jaws of individual patients. Some of their results are summarised in Figure 11.5. The data shown here relate to 229 fixtures in 33 upper jaws and 155 fixtures in 28 lower jaws. The two survival curves indicate clear differences between upper and lower jaw fixture survival.

11.3 META-ANALYSIS

There are many situations in which medical studies done by different investigators have addressed the same or similar questions. In the context of clinical trials, which we will discuss in some detail, these studies may be a group of randomised trials. It

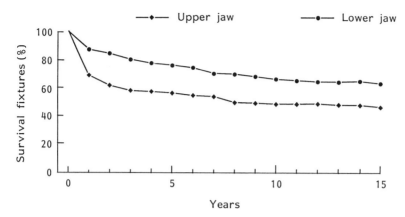

Figure 11.5 Estimated survival functions of stable prosthesis supporting fixtures of the upper and lower jaw (From Eriksson and Adell, 1994 with permission)

is good practice to consider these groups of studies together to assess whether there is evidence of a difference between groups and also to estimate the likely size of this effect. Such a formal quantitative review of all relevant studies is called a meta-analysis or overview.

Meta-analysis can range from one extreme of the combination of a few summary statistics retrieved from published papers, to the other extreme in which every effort is made to identify and collect updated individual subject data from every relevant study (published or unpublished) that has been performed. Stewart and Parmar (1993) give a detailed description of the difference between these two approaches. They demonstrate that the first approach can, in particular for survival data, provide misleading results.

We note that in a survival time context updated data imply that, for example, the current status of any patient alive at the time of reporting the individual trials is requested. In this way the overview will often include more events and longer follow-up than the combined number reported by the trials at their respective times of publication.

We emphasise that meta-analyses of individual patient data aim to include both trials that have been published in the literature and those that, for whatever reason, have not been published. Thus, such an overview aims to summarise all the available evidence relevant to the question.

Example from the literature

The Advanced Ovarian Cancer Trialists' Group (1991) describe the results of all known randomised trials investigating the role of chemotherapy in advanced ovarian cancer. The meta-analysis of these trials included updated survival information from more than 8000 patients. The largest trial amongst these was of 200 patients which, given the current expectations with respect to the magnitude of treatment benefits that are likely to arise in cancer treatment trials, is itself too small for the purpose intended. None of these trials individually had been able to establish the role of chemotherapy.

If there are k randomised trials, each comparing a new treatment, N, with a control or standard treatment, C, then each trial provides an observed number of events in each treatment arm together with the corresponding expected number of events obtained from the logrank test calculations. From these the efficient score (see section 3.9) is

$$U_i = O_{Ci} - E_{Ci} \qquad (11.11)$$

and $i = 1, 2, \ldots, k$. This expression is of the form of the numerator in the exponential part of equation (4.12).

The corresponding variance V_i is equal to that given by equation (4.10). Thus

$$V_i = \sum_t \frac{m_t n_t r_t s_t}{N_t^2(N_t - 1)}. \qquad (11.12)$$

In this way, each trial in the overview provides an estimate of $HR_i = \exp(U_i/V_i)$. An overall estimate of the treatment effect obtained by combining information from all k trials, and which assumes that the true effect does not differ across trials, is given by

$$\log HR_{Av} = \frac{[\sum(\log HR_i/V_i)]}{\sum(1/V_i)}. \qquad (11.13)$$

This averages the HRs obtained from each trial in such a way as also to take account of the relative information provided by each trial. In this way a trial with a large number of events will influence the average more than that which includes few events. This estimate has an SE given by

$$SE(\log HR_{Av}) = \sqrt{[1/\sum(1/V_i)]}. \qquad (11.14)$$

An approximate 95% CI for HR_{Av} is therefore given by

$$\exp\{\log HR_{Av} - 1.96\sqrt{[1/\sum(1/V_i)]}\} \quad \text{to} \quad \exp\{\log HR_{Av} + 1.96\sqrt{[1/\sum(1/V_i)]}\}. \qquad (11.15)$$

We have presented only one approach to combining the information from different but related studies. There are other approaches that may be used. There is no general agreement as to the best approach. Thompson and Pocock (1991) give examples of the different approaches and provide a fuller discussion of these issues.

Example from the literature

Yudkin et al. (1991) conducted a meta-analysis of randomised controlled trials of azathioprine treatment for freedom of relapse in patients with multiple sclerosis. A summary of the results of seven trials at 1 year of follow-up is illustrated in Figure 11.6.

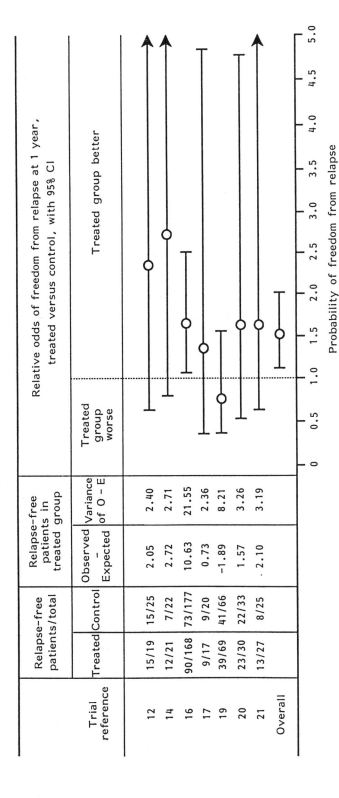

Figure 11.6 The overview analysis of trials of azathioprine for patients with multiple sclerosis (From Yudkin *et al.*, 1991, Overview of aziathioprine treatment in multiple sclerosis, *Lancet* 338, 1051–1055, © by The Lancet Ltd)

At a cursory glance this meta-analysis appears to use survival techniques as it involves survival type measures, notably relapse-free survival. However, the analysis they have conducted reports comparisons at fixed time points only and that is why relative odds (OR) rather than HRs and var(log OR) rather than var(log HR) are used. Nevertheless, their detailed presentation illustrates several important features of a meta analysis as analagous methods of analysis apply. Figure 11.6 shows, for each of the seven trials in this part of their meta-analysis, the estimate of the OR for freedom from relapse at 1-year, together with the associated 95% CI. The analagous efficient score U of equation (11.11) and the analagous variance V of equation (11.12) are also given, together with the number of patients and relapses observed per treatment group. This presentation therefore provides the key elements required for an assessment of the trial results. We note that six of the seven trials have an estimate which indicates a more favourable outcome for the azathioprine-treated group. However, five of these seven have very wide 95% CIs, leaving considerable uncertainty surrounding the result of each trial. Only the largest trial (trial 16) showed an advantage to azathioprine treatment which is significant at the 5% level.

Returning to survival type data, for each individual trial, the null hypothesis is that there is no difference between treatments with respect to survival, i.e. $\log HR_i = 0$ or $HR_i = 1$. Hence, for k trials addressing the same question in a meta-analysis, the combined null hypothesis that the treatment effect is zero in all trials is

$$\log HR_1 = \log HR_2 = \ldots = \log HR_k = 0.$$

If this combined null hypothesis is true, then it can be shown that

$$\chi^2 = \frac{[\sum(\log HR_i/V_i)]^2}{\sum(1/V_i)} \tag{11.16}$$

has a χ^2 distribution with df = 1.

If this combined null hypothesis is rejected this would indicate that at least one of the HRs is different from zero and thus that there is a difference between treatments. However, this does not imply that the difference is a constant for all trials. As a consequence, it is usual to test the homogeneity of treatment effects across studies. This can be done by calculating

$$Q = \sum[(\log HR_i - \log HR_{Av})^2/V_i]. \tag{11.17}$$

Under the null hypothesis of the same, that is homogeneous, treatment differences across the k trials, Q follows a χ^2 distribution with df = (k − 1). It should be noted that this test will only detect large departures from homogeneity. A large value of Q may indicate either that the trials should not be averaged using equation (11.13).

Example from the literature

For the seven trials of azathioprine reported by Yudkin *et al.* (1991) and summarised in Figure 11.6 a test for homogeneity gave Q = 5.17. The df = 7 − 1 = 6 in this case so that from Table T3 we obtain a p-value >0.2. The authors indicate that this is not statistically significant. They also indicate that a test of the combined null hypothesis of no treatment effect gave a p-value <0.01.

11.4 PARAMETRIC MODELLING

We have concentrated in this book on models based on the Cox proportional hazards model. Nevertheless, there are situations in which regression models can be derived as extensions to the exponential or Weibull hazards of chapter 3. For example, in the case of the exponential survival, a model for the parameter λ may be proposed. In such a model the value of the hazard, although constant over time, may vary depending on, for example, particular prognostic features of the patients.

Example from the literature

Feigl and Zelen (1965) examine the influence of white blood cell count (WBC) on the survival of two groups of patients with acute myelogenous leukaemia. The patients, all of whom had died and so there were no censored observations, were first divided into two groups with respect to a characteristic of their white cells, termed AG positive and AG negative. For each AG group they propose a model of the form

$$1/\lambda = \beta_0 + \beta_1 \log \text{WBC}. \tag{11.18}$$

They model $1/\lambda$ rather than λ for technical reasons associated with obtaining maximum likelihood estimates of the regression coefficients.

Here, the individual survival times are assumed to have an exponential distribution of the form of equation (3.3), but with hazard λ depending on the value of the prognostic variable WBC. For the 17 patients who were AG positive, they estimated that $\lambda_{AG+} = 1/(240 - 19.1 \log \text{WBC})$. For those with AG negative $\lambda_{AG-} = 1/(30 - 1.3 \log \text{WBC})$. These both suggest that as WBC increases the hazard also increases. Using these models an AG-positive patient with WBC = 10 000, $\log 10\,000 = 9.2103$ has $\lambda_{AG+} = 1/64.1 = 0.0156$, whereas an AG-negative patient with the same WBC has $\lambda_{AG-} = 1/18.0 = 0.0555$. These give a $\text{HR} = \lambda_{AG-}/\lambda_{AG+} = 0.0555/0.0156 = 3.6$, indicating a worse prognosis for those who are AG negative.

In the case of a Weibull hazard we can derive a model including a potential prognostic factor by

$$\lambda(t; x) = \kappa \lambda (\lambda t)^{\kappa-1} \exp(\beta x). \tag{11.19}$$

Such a model is of the form of that given for the Cox model of equation (6.12) but $\lambda_0(t)$ is now specified in terms of λ and κ which can be estimated. Here x is the value of the covariate for a particular patient and β the associated regression coefficient. This hazard reduces to that of equation (3.13) if $\exp(\beta x) = 0$. This will arise, either if the patient has $x = 0$, a value which corresponds to that of the baseline hazard group, or if the regression coefficient $\beta = 0$. The latter implies the variable under consideration has little or no influence on prognosis.

More details of this model and how it is fitted to data are given by Collett (1994, chapters 4 and 11).

Example from the literature

Byar *et al.* (1979) fitted an extension of equation (11.19) with six covariates to survival data from 500 patients with histologically confirmed thyroid cancer. Their fitted model gave $\lambda = 0.9$ and $\kappa = 0.8$, so that the baseline hazard is $\lambda_0(t) = 0.8 \times 0.9$ $(0.9t)^{(0.8-1)} = 0.74t^{-0.2}$. This is then multiplied by the remainder of the model, which is: $\exp(0.046\ \text{age} - 0.559\ \text{sex} + 0.479\ \text{principal cell type} + 2.049\ \text{anaplastic cell type} + 0.477\ \text{T-category} + 0.679\ \text{metastatic site})$. Here age is treated as a continuous variable; sex was coded 1 for male, 0 for female; there were three cell types requiring two dummy variables with the first set to 1 if principal cell type and 0 otherwise, the second set to 1 if anaplastic and 0 otherwise; T-category was regarded as binary with T_0, T_1 and T_2 in one group with value 0 and T_3 with value 1; finally metastatic sites were non (0), single (1) or multiple (2) and were regarded as an ordered categorical variable.

Table 11.8 A comparison of Weibull and Cox models for the time to develop asthmatic symptoms in workers from seven Norwegian aluminium plants (From Samuelson and Kongerud, 1994 with permission)

variable	Weibull β (SE)	Cox β (SE)
Age	−0.25 (0.16)	−0.29 (0.17)
Sex (M = 1, F = 0)	−0.40 (0.30)	−0.40 (0.27)
Allergy (Y = 1, N = 0)	0.07 (0.37)	0.07 (0.35)
Asthma in family (Y = 1, N = 0)	0.39 (0.26)	0.39 (0.24)
Previous exposure (Y = 1, N = 0)	0.60 (0.24)	0.60 (0.23)
Never smoker	0	0
Ex-smoker	1.43 (0.66)	1.42 (0.55)
Light smoker	0.55 (0.28)	0.55 (0.27)
Heavy smoker	1.04 (0.31)	1.01 (0.27)
Soederberg oven	0	0
Prebake oven	0.40 (0.26)	0.42 (0.27)
Rotation	0.93 (0.32)	0.94 (0.31)
Low fluoride	0	0
Medium fluoride	1.37 (0.39)	1.36 (0.38)
High fluoride	2.28 (0.47)	2.25 (0.48)
Fluoride not classified	0.72 (0.31)	0.75 (0.29)

Example from the literature

A comparison of the Cox proportional hazards model and a Weibull model both including covariates is given by Samuelsen and Kongerud (1994). They describe a study of workers in seven Norwegian aluminium plants in which information on the time to develop asthmatic symptoms in more than 1000 new employees is collected. The two models arising from their analyses are summarised in Table 11.8. From these it is very clear that the results obtained via both models are very similar.

11.5 SEQUENTIAL TRIALS

In the sample size calculations of chapter 10 we described the design of trials in which a fixed number of events are to be observed in the trial. This in turn requires a fixed number of patients to be recruited to the trial. The appropriate number of patients is then recruited and the analysis performed and trial results reported once the prerequisite number of events is observed.

An alternative is to use a sequential design. With such a design, the data are analysed as they accumulate and according to a pre-specified schedule. Such 'interim' analyses may permit, for example, an early closure to patient recruitment, if a clear advantage to one group is observed.

Details of certain sequential designs, as they apply to survival time applications,

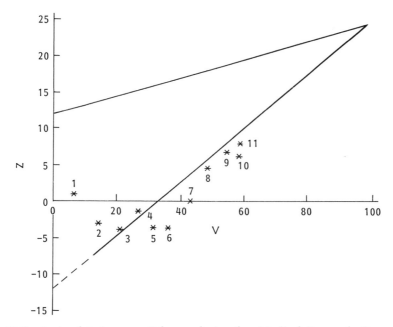

Figure 11.7 A simulated sequential reanalysis of a Medical Research Council trial of maintenance versus non-maintenance chemotherapy in the management of small cell lung cancer (modified from Donaldson *et al.*, 1993, by permission of The Macmillan Press Ltd)

are given in the book by Whitehead (1992). In brief, sequential designs involve specifying boundaries (see Figure 11.7) and the interim analyses are summarised as successive points on a graphical plot of $Z(= U/V)$ against the variance, V, where U, the efficient score, and V are defined by equations (11.10) and (11.12), as we have indicated earlier in this chapter when describing meta-analyses. However, in a sequential trial they are calculated from all the data available at each successive interim analysis. We note that at each successive interim analysis the value of V, which depends on the number of events observed, increases. If a point (V, Z) at one of the interim analyses crosses a boundary then this indicates that there may be persuasive evidence concerning relative efficacy of the therapies under test and the recruitment of further patients may not be necessary.

Note, however, in contrast to V, the efficient score U can increase or decrease in magnitude and can change sign from analysis to analysis.

Example from the literature

Donaldson et al. (1993) describe a reanalysis of a completed and published fixed-sample size clinical trial in 265 patients with small cell lung cancer. In this reanalysis a sequential design that may have been appropriate for such a trial was first specified. The accumulated data as they would have appeared at successive interim analyses were then extracted from the trial data base and analysed. Figure 11.7 shows the plot of 11 such interim analyses which mimic, at least in the earlier points, what would have occurred had this trial been truly sequential.

The plot indicates that the fifth such analysis would have given a point outside the boundary. In brief, such a point would indicate that there may be sufficient evidence from the trial data to terminate further recruitment at this stage. Readers are referred to the original article and also one by Whitehead (1993) for more precise details.

References

Aboulker JP and Swart AM (1993). Preliminary analysis of the Concorde Trial. *Lancet*, **341**, 889–890. [1]

Advanced Ovarian Cancer Trialists Group (1991). Chemotherapy in advanced ovarian cancer: an overview of randomised clinical trials. *British Medical Journal*, **303**, 884–893. [11]

Altman DG (1991). *Practical Statistics for Medical Research*. Chapman & Hall, London. [1, 5]

Altman DG and de Stavola BL (1994). Practical problems in fitting a proportional hazards model to data with updated measurements of the covariates. *Statistics in Medicine*, **13**, 301–341. [8]

Azen SP, Roy S, Pike MC and Casagrande J (1976). Some suggested improvements to current statistical methods for analysing contraceptive efficacy. *Journal of Chronic Diseases*, **29**, 649–666. [11]

Bland M (1987). *An Introduction to Medical Statistics*. Oxford University Press, Oxford. [1]

Bleehen NM and Stenning SP on behalf of the Medical Research Council Brain Tumour Working Party (1991). A Medical Research Council trial of two radiotherapy doses in the treatment of grades 3 and 4 astrocytoma. *British Journal of Cancer*, **64**, 769–774. [2, 6, 9]

Breslow NE and Day NE (1980). *Statistical Methods in Cancer Research. Volume 1: The Analysis of Case–Control Studies*. IARC Scientific Publications, Lyon. [1]

Breslow NE and Day NE (1987). *Statistical Methods in Cancer Research. Volume 2: The Design and Analysis of Cohort Studies*. IARC Scientific Publications, Lyon. [1]

Byar DP, Green SB, Dor P, Williams ED, Colon J, van Gilse HA, Mayer M, Sylvester RJ and Van Glabbeke M (1979). A prognostic index for thyroid carcinoma. A study of the EORTC Thyroid Cancer Cooperative Group. *European Journal of Cancer*, **15**, 1033–1041. [11]

Campbell MJ and Machin D (1993). *Medical Statistics: A Commonsense Approach* (2nd edn). Wiley, Chichester. [1, 4]

Chant ADB, Turner DTL and Machin D (1983). Metronidazole v ampicillin: differing effects on the post-operative recovery. *Annals of the Royal College of Surgeons of England*, **66**, 96–97. [10]

Cheingsong-Popov R, Panagiotidi C, Bowcock S, Aronstam A, Wadsworth J and Weber J (1991). Relation between humoral responses to HIV gag and end proteins at seroconversion and clinical outcome of HIV infection. *British Medical Journal*, **302**, 23–26. [4]

Christensen E (1987). Multivariate survival analysis using Cox's regression model. *Hepatology*, **7**, 1346–1358. [1]

Clayton D and Hills M (1993). *Statistical Models in Epidemiology*. Oxford University Press, Oxford. [1]

Collett D (1994). *Modelling Survival Data in Medical Research*. Chapman & Hall, London. [1, 10]

COMPACT Steering Committee (1991). Improving the quality of data in clinical trials in cancer. *British Journal of Cancer*, 63, 412–415. [1]

Cox DR (1972). Regression models and life tables (with discussion). *Journal of the Royal Statistical Society*, B34, 187–220. [1, 6]

Cox DR and Oakes D (1984). *Analysis of Survival Data*. Chapman & Hall, London. [1]

Donaldson AN, Whitehead J, Stephens R and Machin D (1993). A simulated sequential analysis based on data from two MRC trials. *British Journal of Cancer*, 68, 1171–1178. [11]

Eriksson B and Adell R (1994). On the analysis of life-tables for dependent observations. *Statistics in Medicine*, 13, 43–51. [11]

Familiari L, Postorino S, Turiano S and Luzza G (1981). Comparison of pirenzepine and trithiozine with placebo in treatment of peptic ulcer. *Clinical Trials Journal*, 18, 363–368. [1]

Farewell VT (1979). An application of Cox's proportional hazards model to multiple infection data. *Applied Statistics*, 28, 136–143. [8]

Farley TMM (1986). Life-table methods for contraceptive research. *Statistics in Medicine*, 5, 475–489. [11]

Farley TMM, Rosenberg MJ, Rowe PJ, Chen J-H and Meirik O (1992). Intrauterine devices and pelvic inflammatory disease: an international perspective. *Lancet*, 339, 785–788. [2]

Feigl P and Zelen M (1965). Estimation of exponential survival probabilities with concomitant information. *Biometrics*, 21, 826–838. [11]

Fisher B, Anderson S, Fisher ER, Redmond C, Wickerham DL, Wolmark N, Mamounas EP, Deutsch M and Margolese R (1991). Significance of ipsilateral breast tumour recurrence after lumpectomy. *Lancet*, 338, 327–331. [2, 6, 8]

France LA, Lewis JA and Kay R (1991). The analysis of failure time data in crossover studies. *Statistics in Medicine*, 10, 1099–1113. [4, 11]

Freedman LS (1982). Tables of the number of patients required in clinical trials using the logrank test. *Statistics in Medicine*, 1, 121–129. [10]

Galloe AM, Rasmussen HS, Jorgensen LN, Aurup P, Balslov S, Cintin C, Graudal N and McNair P (1993). Influence of oral magnesium supplementation on cardiac events among survivors of an acute myocardial infarction. *British Medical Journal*, 307, 585–587. [1]

Gardner MJ and Altman DG (eds) (1989). *Statistics with Confidence*. British Medical Association, London. [1]

Gerhartz HH, Engelhard M, Meusers P, Brittinger G, Wilmanns W, Schlimok G, Mueller P, Huhn D, Musch R, Siegert W, Gerhartz D, Harlapp JH, Thiel E, Huber C, Peschi C, Spann W, Emmerich B, Schadek C, Westerhausen M, Pees H-W, Radtke H, Engert A, Terhardt E, Schick H, Binder T, Fuchs R, Hasford J, Brandmaier R, Stern AC, Jones TC, Ehrlich HJ, Stein H, Parwaresch M, Tiemann M and Lennert K (1993). Randomized, double-blind, placebo-controlled, phase III study of recombinant human granulocyte–macrophage colony-stimulating factor as adjunct to induction treatment of high-grade malignant non-Hodgkin's lymphomas. *Blood*, 82, 2329–2339. [10]

Gray R, James R, Mossman J and Stenning SP (1991) On behalf of the ISK Coordinating Committee on Cancer Research (UKCCCR) Colorectal Cancer Subcommittee. Axis: a suitable case for treatment. *British Journal of Cancer*, 63, 841–845. [6]

Greenwood M (1926). *The Natural Duration of Cancer*. Reports of Public Health and Medical Subjects, 33. HMSO, London. [2]

Gross AJ and Clark VA (1975). *Survival Distributions: Reliability Applications in the Biomedical Sciences*. Wiley, New York. [1]

Gross AJ and Lam CF (1981). Paired observations from a survival distribution. *Biometrics*, 37, 505–511. [11]

Hankey GJ, Slattery JM and Warlow CP (1991). Prognosis and prognostic factors of retinal infarction: a prospective cohort study. *British Medical Journal*, 302, 499–504. [2]

Harris EK and Albert A (1991). *Survivorship Analysis for Clinical Studies*. Marcel Dekker, New York. [2]

Higgens JE and Wilkens LR (1985). Statistical comparison of Pearl rates. *American Journal of Obstetrics and Gynecology*, 151, 656–659. [11]

Kalbfleisch JD and Prentice RL (1980). *The Statistical Analysis of Failure Time Data*. Wiley, New York. [1]

Khawaja HT, Campbell MJ and Weaver PC (1988). Effect of transdermal glyceryl trinitrate on the survival of peripheral intravenous infusions: a double-blind prospective clinical study. *British Journal of Surgery*, 75, 1212–1215. [2]

Lee ET (1992). *Statistical Methods for Survival Data Analysis* (2nd edn). Wiley, New York. [1, 2]

Lentner G (ed.) (1991). *Geigy Scientific Tables. 2: Introduction to Statistics, Statistical Tables and Mathematical Formulae*. Ciba-Geigy, Basle, Switzerland. [2]

Leonard RCF, Hayward RL, Prescott RJ and Wang JX (1991). The identification of discrete prognostic groups in low-grade non-Hodgkin's lymphoma. *Annals of Oncology*, 2, 655–662. [9]

Machin D and Campbell MJ (1987). *Statistical Tables for the Design of Clinical Trials*. Blackwell Scientific Publications, Oxford. [1, 10]

Mackie RM, Bufalino R, Morabito A, Sutherland C and Cascinelli N for the World Health Organization Melanoma Programme (1991). Lack of effect of pregnancy on outcome of melanoma. *Lancet*, 337, 653–655. [8]

Mantel N and Haenszel W (1959). Statistical aspects of the analysis of data from retrospective studies of disease. *Journal of the National Cancer Institute*, 22, 719–748. [1]

Mayo NE, Korner-Bitensky NA and Becker R (1991). Recovery time at independent function post-stroke. *American Journal of Physical Medicine and Rehabilitation*, 70, 5–12. [1, 6]

McDiarmid T, Burns PN, Lewith GT and Machin D (1985). Ultrasound and the treatment of pressure sores: preliminary study. *Physiotherapy*, 71, 66–70. [4]

McIllmurray MB and Turkie W (1987). Controlled trial of γ linolenic acid in Dukes' C colorectal cancer. *British Medical Journal*, 294, 1260; 295, 475. [2, 3]

Medical Research Council Brain Tumour Working Party (1990). Prognostic factors for malignant glioma: development of a prognostic index. *Journal of Neuro-Oncology*, 9, 47–55. [9]

Medical Research Council Lung Cancer Working Party (1989a). Survival, adverse reactions and quality of life during combination chemotherapy compared with selective palliative treatment for small-cell lung cancer. *Respiratory Medicine*, 83, 51–58. [6]

Medical Research Council Lung Cancer Working Party (1989b). Controlled trial of twelve versus six courses of chemotherapy in the treatment of small-cell lung cancer. *British Journal of Cancer*, 59, 584–590. [6]

Medical Research Council Lung Cancer Working Party (1991). Inoperable non-small-cell lung cancer (NSCLC): a Medical Research Council randomised trial of palliative radiotherapy with two fractions or ten fractions. *British Journal of Cancer*, 63, 265–270. [6]

Medical Research Council Lung Cancer Working Party (1992). A Medical Research Council (MRC) randomised trial of palliative radiotherapy with two fractions or a single fraction in patients with inoperable non-small-cell lung cancer (NSCLC) and poor performance status. *British Journal of Cancer*, 65, 934–941. [6]

Medical Research Council Lung Cancer Working Party (1993). A randomised trial of 3 or 6 courses of etoposide, cyclophosphamide, methotrexate and vincristine, or 6 courses of etoposide and ifosfamide in small-cell lung cancer (SCLC). I: Survival and prognostic factors. *British Journal of Cancer*, 68, 1150–1156. [6, 8]

Medical Research Council Working Party on Advanced Carcinoma of the Cervix (1993). A trial of Ro 03–8799 (pimonidazole) in carcinoma of the uterine cervix: an interim report from the Medical Research Council Working Party on advanced carcinoma of the cervix. *Radiotherapy and Oncology*, 26, 93–103. [4, 5]

Medical Research Council Working Party on Misonidazole in Gliomas (1983). A study of the effect of misonidazole in conjunction with radiotherapy for the treatment of grades 3 and 4 astrocytomas. *British Journal of Radiology*, 56, 673–682. [4, 6, 7, 9]

Meng CD, Zhu JC, Chen ZW, Wong LT, Zhang GY, Hu YZ, Ding JH, Wang XH, Qian SZ, Wang C, Machin D, Pinol A and Waikes GMH (1988). Recovery of sperm production following the cessation of gossypol treatment: a two centre study in China. *International Journal of Andrology*, 11, 1–11.   [1, 6]

Moffatt CJ, Franks PJ, Oldroyd M, Bosanquet N, Brown P, Greenhalgh RM and McCollum CN. (1992). Community clinics for leg ulcers and impact on healing. *British Medical Journal*, 305, 1389–1392.   [2]

Mufti GJ, Stevens JR, Oscier DG, Hamblin TJ and Machin D (1985). Myelodysplastic syndromes: a scoring system with prognostic significance. *British Journal of Haematology*, 59, 425–433.   [4, 5]

Multicenter Study Group (1980). Long-term oral acetylcysteine in chronic bronchitis: a double-blind controlled study. *European Journal of Respiratory Diseases*, 51, Suppl. 111, 93–108.   [1]

Nash TP, Williams JD, Machin D (1990). TENS: does the type of stimulus really matter? *Pain Clinic*, 3, 161–168.   [4, 5]

Nolan T, Debelle G, Oberklaid F and Coffey C (1991). Randomised trials of laxatives in treatment of childhood encopresis. *Lancet*, 338, 523–527.   [4]

Packer M, Carver JR, Rodeheffer RJ, Ivanhoe RJ, DiBianco R, Zeldis SM, Hendrix GH, Bommer WJ, Elkayam U, Kukin ML, Mallis GL, Sollano A, Shannon J, Tandon PK and DeMets DL for the PROMISE Study Research Group (1991). Effect of oral milrinone on mortality in severe chronic heart failure. *New England Journal of Medicine*, 325, 1468–1475.   [1, 4]

Parmar MKB and Machin D (1993). Monitoring clinical trials: experience of, and proposals under consideration by, the Cancer Therapy Committee of the British Medical Research Council. *Statistics in Medicine*, 12, 497–504.   [4]

Parmar MKB, Spiegelhalter DJ and Freedman LS (1994). The CHART trials: Bayesian design and monitoring in practice. *Statistics in Medicine*, 13, 1297–1312.   [10]

Peto J (1984). The calculation and interpretation of survival curves. In: Buyse ME, Staquet MJ and Sylvester RJ (eds), *Cancer Clinical Trials: Methods and Practice*. Oxford University Press, Oxford, pp. 361–380.   [2]

Peto R, Pike MC, Armitage P, Breslow NE, Cox DR, Howard SV, Mantel N, MacPherson K, Peto J and Smith PG (1976). Design and analysis of randomised clinical trials requiring prolonged observation of each patient. I: Introduction and design. *British Journal of Cancer*, 34, 585–612.   [1]

Peto R, Pike MC, Armitage P, Breslow NE, Cox DR, Howard SV, Mantel N, MacPherson K, Peto J and Smith PG (1977). Design and analysis of randomised clinical trials requiring prolonged observation of each patient. II: Analysis and examples. *British Journal of Cancer*, 35, 1–39.   [1]

Pocock SJ (1983). *Clinical Trials: A Practical Approach*. Wiley, Chichester.   [1]

RISC Group (1990). Risk of myocardial infarction and death during treatment with low dose aspirin and intravenous heparin in men with unstable coronary artery disease. *Lancet*, 336, 827–830.   [5, 6]

Rothman KJ (1978). Estimation of confidence limits for the cumulative probability of survival in life table analysis. *Journal of Chronic Diseases*, 31, 557–560.   [2]

Samanta A, Roy S and Woods KL (1991). Gold therapy in rheumatoid arthritis. *Lancet*, 338, 642.   [2]

Samuelsen SO and Kongerud J (1994). Interval censoring in longitudinal data of respiratory symptoms in aluminium pot room workers. *Statistics in Medicine*, 13, 1771–1780.   [11]

Senn S (1993). *Crossover Trials in Clinical Research*. Wiley, Chichester.   [11]

Shuster JJ (1991). Median follow-up in clinical trials. *Journal of Clinical Oncology*, 9, 191–192.   [2]

Simon R and Altman DG (1994). Statistical aspects of prognostic factor studies in oncology. *British Journal of Cancer*, 69, 979–985.   [6, 7]

Stephens RJ, Girling DJ and Machin D (1994). Can patients at risk from death during treatment for small cell lung cancer be identified? *Lung Cancer*, 11, 259–274.   [2]

Stewart LS and Parmar MKB (1993) Meta-analysis of the literature or individual patient data: is there a difference? *Lancet*, **341**, 418–422. [11]

Thompson SG and Pocock SJ (1991) Can meta-analyses be trusted? *Lancet*, **338**, 1127–1130. [11]

Tibsharani R (1982). A plain man's guide to the proportional hazards model. *Clinical Investigative Medicine*, **5**, 63–68. [1]

Turnbull BW, Brown BW Jr and Hu M (1974). Survivorship analysis of heart transplant data. *Journal of the American Statistical Association*, **69**, 74–86. [1, 2]

Umen AJ and Le CT (1986). Prognostic factors, models and related statistical problems in the survival of end-stage renal disease patients on hemodialysis. *Statistics in Medicine*, **5**, 637–652. [7]

Valerius NH, Koch C and Hoiby N (1991). Prevention of chronic *Pseudomonas aeruginosa* colonisation in cystic fibrosis by early treatment. *Lancet*, **338**, 725–726. [10]

Valsecchi MG and Marubini E (1995) *Analysing Survival Data from Clinical Trials and Observational Studies*. Wiley, Chichester. [1]

Van Griensven GJP, Boucher EC, Roos M and Coutinho RA (1991). Expansion of AIDS case definition. *Lancet*, **338**, 1012–1013. [2]

Vessey M, Doll R, Peto R, Johnson B and Wiggins P (1976). A long-term follow-up study of women using different methods of contraception—an interim report. *Journal of Biosocial Science*, **8**, 373–427. [11]

Wheeler JG, Machin D, Campbell MJ, Stephens RJ, Bleehen NM and Girling DJ for the Medical Research Council Lung Cancer Working Party (1994). Does clinical experience with a treatment regimen affect survival of lung cancer patients? An analysis based on consecutive randomised trials of the Medical Research Council in small cell and non-small cell tumours. *Clinical Oncology*, **6**, 81–90. [6]

Whitehead J (1992). *The Design and Analysis of Sequential Clinical Trials* (2nd edn). Ellis Horwood, New York. [11]

Whitehead J (1993). Interim analyses and stopping rules in cancer clinical trials. *British Journal of Cancer*, **68**, 1179–1185. [11]

Whitehead J and Dorse C (1988). Prospective epidemiological studies involving paired organs. *Statistics in Medicine*, **7**, 619–625. [11]

World Health Organization Task Force on Long-acting Systemic Agents for Fertility Regulation (1986). A multicentred Phase III comparative clinical trial of depot-medroxyprogesterone acetate given three-monthly at doses of 100 mg or 150 mg. I: Contraceptive efficacy and side effects. *Contraception*, **34**, 223–260. [11]

World Health Organization Task Force on Long-acting Systemic Agents for Fertility Regulation. Special Programme of Research, Development and Research training in Human Reproduction (1988). A multicentred phase III comparative study of two hormonal contraceptive preparations given once-a-month by intramuscular injections. I: Contraceptive efficacy and side effects. *Contraception*, **37**, 1–20. [4]

World Health Organization Task Force on Long-acting Systemic Agents for Fertility Regulation (1990). Microdose intravaginal levenorgestrel contraception: a multicentre clinical trial. III. The relationship between pregnancy rate and body weight. *Contraception*, **41**, 143–150. [5, 7]

World Health Organization Task Force for the Regulation of Male Fertility (1990). Contraceptive efficacy of testosterone-induced azoospermia in normal men. *Lancet*, **336**, 955–959. [11]

Yudkin PL, Ellison GW, Ghezzi A, Goodkin DE, Hughes RAC, McPherson K, Mertin J and Milanese C (1991). Overview of aziathioprine treatment in multiple sclerosis. *Lancet*, **338**, 1051–1055. [11]

Statistical Tables

Table T1   The Normal distribution
The value tabulated is the probability, α, that a random variable, Normally distributed with mean zero and standard deviation one will be greater than z or less than −z.

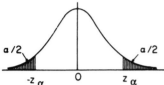

z	0.00	0.01	0.02	0.03	0.04	0.05	0.06	0.07	0.08	0.09
0.00	1.0000	0.9920	0.9840	0.9761	0.9681	0.9601	0.9522	0.9442	0.9362	0.9283
0.10	0.9203	0.9124	0.9045	0.8966	0.8887	0.8808	0.8729	0.8650	0.8572	0.8493
0.20	0.8415	0.8337	0.8259	0.8181	0.8103	0.8026	0.7949	0.7872	0.7795	0.7718
0.30	0.7642	0.7566	0.7490	0.7414	0.7339	0.7263	0.7188	0.7114	0.7039	0.6965
0.40	0.6892	0.6818	0.6745	0.6672	0.6599	0.6527	0.6455	0.6384	0.6312	0.6241
0.50	0.6171	0.6101	0.6031	0.5961	0.5892	0.5823	0.5755	0.5687	0.5619	0.5522
0.60	0.5485	0.5419	0.5353	0.5287	0.5222	0.5157	0.5093	0.5029	0.4965	0.4902
0.70	0.4839	0.4777	0.4715	0.4654	0.4593	0.4533	0.4473	0.4413	0.4354	0.4295
0.80	0.4237	0.4179	0.4122	0.4065	0.4009	0.3953	0.3898	0.3843	0.3789	0.3735
0.90	0.3681	0.3628	0.3576	0.3524	0.3472	0.3421	0.3371	0.3320	0.3271	0.3222
1.00	0.3173	0.3125	0.3077	0.3030	0.2983	0.2937	0.2891	0.2846	0.2801	0.2757

z	0.00	0.01	0.02	0.03	0.04	0.05	0.06	0.07	0.08	0.09
1.10	0.3173	0.3125	0.3077	0.3030	0.2983	0.2937	0.2891	0.2846	0.2801	0.2757
1.10	0.2713	0.2670	0.2627	0.2585	0.2543	0.2501	0.2460	0.2420	0.2380	0.2340
1.20	0.2301	0.2263	0.2225	0.2187	0.2150	0.2113	0.2077	0.2041	0.2005	0.1971
1.30	0.1936	0.1902	0.1868	0.1835	0.1802	0.1770	0.1738	0.1707	0.1676	0.1645
1.40	0.1615	0.1585	0.1556	0.1527	0.1499	0.1471	0.1443	0.1416	0.1389	0.1362
1.50	0.1336	0.1310	0.1285	0.1260	0.1236	0.1211	0.1188	0.1164	0.1141	0.1118
1.60	0.1096	0.1074	0.1052	0.1031	0.1010	0.0989	0.0969	0.0949	0.0930	0.0910
1.70	0.0891	0.0873	0.0854	0.0836	0.0819	0.0801	0.0784	0.0767	0.0751	0.0735
1.80	0.0719	0.0703	0.0688	0.0672	0.0658	0.0643	0.0629	0.0615	0.0601	0.0588
1.90	0.0574	0.0561	0.0549	0.0536	0.0524	0.0512	0.0500	0.0488	0.0477	0.0466
2.00	0.0455	0.0444	0.0434	0.0424	0.0414	0.0404	0.0394	0.0385	0.0375	0.0366

z	0.00	0.01	0.02	0.03	0.04	0.05	0.06	0.07	0.08	0.09
2.00	0.0455	0.0444	0.0434	0.0424	0.0414	0.0404	0.0394	0.0385	0.0375	0.0366
2.10	0.0357	0.0349	0.0340	0.0332	0.0324	0.0316	0.0308	0.0300	0.0293	0.0285
2.20	0.0278	0.0271	0.0264	0.0257	0.0251	0.0244	0.0238	0.0232	0.0226	0.0220
2.30	0.0214	0.0209	0.0203	0.0198	0.0193	0.0188	0.0183	0.0178	0.0173	0.0168
2.40	0.0164	0.0160	0.0155	0.0151	0.0147	0.0143	0.0139	0.0135	0.0131	0.0128
2.50	0.0124	0.0121	0.0117	0.0114	0.0111	0.0108	0.0105	0.0102	0.0099	0.0096
2.60	0.0093	0.0091	0.0088	0.0085	0.0083	0.0080	0.0078	0.0076	0.0074	0.0071
2.70	0.0069	0.0067	0.0065	0.0063	0.0061	0.0060	0.0058	0.0056	0.0054	0.0053
2.80	0.0051	0.0050	0.0048	0.0047	0.0045	0.0044	0.0042	0.0041	0.0040	0.0039
2.90	0.0037	0.0036	0.0035	0.0034	0.0033	0.0032	0.0031	0.0030	0.0029	0.0028
3.00	0.0027	0.0026	0.0025	0.0024	0.0024	0.0023	0.0022	0.0021	0.0021	0.0020

Table T2 Percentage points of the
Normal distribution

1-sided		2-sided
α	z	α
0.0005	3.2905	0.0010
0.0025	2.8070	0.0050
0.0050	2.5758	0.0100
0.0100	2.3263	0.0200
0.0125	2.2414	0.0250
0.0250	1.9600	0.0500
0.0500	1.6449	0.1000
0.1000	1.2816	0.2000
0.1500	1.0364	0.3000
0.2000	0.8416	0.4000
0.2500	0.6745	0.5000
0.3000	0.5244	0.6000
0.3500	0.3853	0.7000
0.4000	0.2533	0.8000

Table T3 The χ^2 distribution

The value tabulated is $\chi^2(\alpha)$, such as that if X is distributed as a χ^2 with df degrees of freedom, then α is the probability that $X \geq \chi^2$.

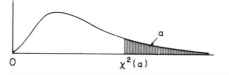

$$0 \qquad \chi^2(a)$$

					α				
	0.2	0.1	0.05	0.04	0.03	0.02	0.01	0.001	0.0005
df = 1	1.64	2.71	3.84	4.22	4.71	5.41	6.63	10.83	12.12
2	3.22	4.61	5.99	6.44	7.01	7.82	9.21	13.82	15.20
3	4.64	6.25	7.81	8.31	8.95	9.84	11.34	16.27	17.73
4	5.99	7.78	9.49	10.03	10.71	11.67	13.28	18.47	20.00
5	7.29	9.24	11.07	11.64	12.37	13.39	15.09	20.52	22.11
6	8.56	10.64	12.59	13.20	13.97	15.03	16.81	22.46	24.10
7	9.80	12.02	14.07	14.70	15.51	16.62	18.48	24.32	26.02
8	11.03	13.36	15.51	16.17	17.01	18.17	20.09	26.13	27.87
9	12.24	14.68	16.92	17.61	18.48	19.68	21.67	27.88	29.67
10	13.44	15.99	18.31	19.02	19.92	21.16	23.21	29.59	31.42
11	14.63	17.28	19.68	20.41	21.34	22.62	24.73	31.26	33.14
12	15.81	18.55	21.03	21.79	22.74	24.05	26.22	32.91	34.82
13	16.98	19.81	22.36	23.14	24.12	25.47	27.69	34.53	36.48
14	18.15	21.06	23.68	24.49	25.49	26.87	29.14	36.12	38.11
15	19.31	22.31	25.00	25.82	26.85	28.26	30.58	37.70	39.72
16	20.47	23.54	26.30	27.14	28.19	29.63	32.00	39.25	41.31
17	21.61	24.77	27.59	28.45	29.52	31.00	33.41	40.79	42.88
18	22.76	25.99	28.87	29.75	30.84	32.35	34.81	42.31	44.43
19	23.90	27.20	30.14	31.04	32.16	33.69	36.19	43.82	45.97
20	25.04	28.41	31.41	32.32	33.46	35.02	37.57	45.32	47.50
21	26.17	29.61	32.67	33.60	34.75	36.34	38.91	47.00	49.01
22	27.30	30.81	33.92	34.87	36.04	37.65	40.32	48.41	50.51
23	28.43	32.01	35.18	36.13	37.33	38.97	41.61	49.81	52.00
24	29.55	33.19	36.41	37.39	38.62	40.26	43.02	51.22	53.48
25	30.67	34.38	37.65	38.65	39.88	41.55	44.30	52.63	54.95
26	31.79	35.56	38.88	39.88	41.14	42.84	45.65	54.03	56.41
27	32.91	36.74	40.12	41.14	42.40	44.13	47.00	55.44	57.86
28	34.03	37.92	41.35	42.37	43.66	45.42	48.29	56.84	59.30
29	35.14	39.09	42.56	43.60	44.92	46.71	49.58	58.25	60.73
30	36.25	40.25	43.78	44.83	46.15	47.97	50.87	59.66	62.16

Table T4 The total number of patients required to detect an improvement $\delta = (\pi_T - \pi_C)$ in survival over the survival rate of the standard therapy π_C, when $\alpha = 0.05$ and power $1 - \beta = 0.8$ (upper figure) and $1 - \beta = 0.9$ (lower figure)

π_C	δ 0.05	0.10	0.15	0.20	0.25	0.30	0.35	0.40	0.45	0.50
0.05	498	174	100	70	54	44	38	32	30	26
	664	232	134	92	72	58	50	44	38	36
0.10	964	296	156	102	74	58	48	40	36	32
	1290	396	208	136	98	76	64	54	46	42
0.15	1416	406	204	128	90	68	56	46	40	34
	1894	544	272	170	120	92	74	62	52	46
0.20	1828	506	246	150	104	78	62	50	42	36
	2446	676	328	200	138	104	82	66	56	48
0.25	2188	590	280	168	114	84	66	64	44	38
	2928	788	376	224	152	112	88	70	60	50
0.30	2488	658	308	182	122	90	68	56	46	40
	3330	880	412	244	164	118	92	74	60	52
0.35	2724	710	328	192	128	90	70	56	46	40
	3648	950	438	256	170	122	94	74	60	52
0.40	2896	744	340	196	130	92	70	56	46	38
	3876	996	454	262	172	124	94	74	60	50
0.45	3000	762	344	198	128	92	68	54	44	38
	4014	1020	460	264	172	122	92	72	58	48
0.50	3034	764	342	194	126	88	66	52	42	
	4062	1020	456	258	166	116	88	68	56	
0.55	3002	746	330	186	120	84	62	48		
	4018	998	442	248	158	110	82	64		
0.60	2900	714	312	174	110	76	56			
	3882	954	418	232	146	102	74			
0.65	2730	664	286	158	100	68				
	3654	886	382	210	132	90				
0.70	2494	596	254	138	86					
	3338	796	338	182	112					
0.75	2190	512	214	114						
	2930	684	284	150						
0.80	1822	414	168							
	2436	552	222							
0.85	1388	300								
	1854	398								
0.90	892									
	1190									

Statistical and Mathematical Symbols

The appropriate chapters in which the principal symbols are first defined are given in square brackets. Some symbols are used for more than one purpose. Subscript labels are often added to the basic characters listed below depending on the context.

α Test size, significance level or probability of a type I error   [1]

β Probability of a type II error; $1 - \beta$ corresponds to the power   [1]

γ Regression coefficient for a dummy variable in a Cox model. Also used with various subscripts depending on the context   [6]

       Regression coefficient for a time-dependent variable in a Cox model   [8]

δ A pre-specified difference between two means, proportions or survival rates   [1]

       The true difference between two means, proportions or survival rates   [1]

Δ A pre-specified value of the hazard ratio   [10]

$\Delta\tau$ A short interval of time   [2]

λ The constant hazard   [3]

$\lambda_0(t)$ The hazard function   [3]

       The baseline hazard in a Cox model   [6]

$\lambda(t)$ The hazard in a Cox model   [6]

κ The shape parameter of a Weibull distribution   [3]

μ Population mean of a group   [1]

π Proportion of individuals having a particular attribute in a population   [1]

Π	Denotes 'the product of'	[2]
Σ	Denotes 'the sum of'	[1]
$\int$	The integral sign	[2]
ϕ	Ratio of the number of subjects in two treatment groups	[10]
$\phi(t)$	Probability density function of a distribution	[2]
χ^2	Chi-squared test	[1]
χ^2_G	The Gehan, Wilcoxon or Breslow test statistic	[4]
$\chi^2_{Logrank}$	Logrank test statistic	[4]
χ^2_{MH}	The Mantel–Haenszel test statistic	[4]
χ^2_{MHw}	The weighted Mantel–Haenszel test statistic	[4]
χ^2_{PP}	The Peto–Prentice test statistic	[4]
χ^2_{TW}	The Tarone–Ware test statistic	[4]
χ^2_{Trend}	The chi-squared test for trend with $df = 1$	[5]
a	Intercept of a linear regression line	[3]
b	Slope of a linear regression line	[3]
	Estimate of regression coefficient in a Cox model	[6]
CI	Confidence interval	[1]
c_j	Number of censored observations in interval j	[2]
d	Number of deaths	[2]
df	Degrees of freedom	[1]
d_t	Number of deaths at time t	[2]
e	The base of natural logarithms $e = 2.71828\ldots$	[1]
exp	The exponential function, denoting the inverse procedure to taking natural logarithms	[1]
E	The expected number of events	[1]
	The number of events required to be observed in a study	[10]
f	Total follow-up or exposure time of dead patients	[2]
F	Total follow-up or exposure time for alive patients	[2]
g	Estimate of regression coefficient of a dummy variable in a Cox model	[6]
	Estimate of regression coefficient of a time-dependent variable in a Cox model	[8]
G	Number of groups	[5]
h	Hazard rate	[2]
h(t)	The hazard function	[2]
	The relative hazard	[6]
HR	Hazard ratio	[1]
H_0	The null hypothesis	[1]
H_A	The alternative hypothesis	[1,10]
l	The likelihood	[1]
L	The log likelihood	[1]
LR	Likelihood ratio	[1]
log	Logarithms to the base e	[1]
M	Median survival time	[2]
n, N	Number of observations or sample size	[1]
n_t	Number alive at time t	[2]

O	Observed number of events [1]
OR	Odds ratio [1]
p	Observed proportion of individuals with a particular attribute in a sample [1]
	p-value. The probability of the data, or some more extreme data, arising by chance when the null hypothesis is true [1]
p_t	Conditional probability of surviving day t given survival to day $t-1$ [2]
PI	Prognostic index [9]
PR	Pearl rate [11]
RR	Relative risk [1]
R_t	Total number at risk at time t [4]
S	The score statistic [6]
	Score derived in calculating a prognostic index [9]
SD	Standard deviation [1]
SE	Standard error [1]
S(t)	Survival function [2]
S(t; x)	Survival function, the value of which may depend on the variable x [6]
$S_{Actuarial}(t)$	Actuarial estimate of the survival function [2]
t	Survival time [2]
T+	Censored survival time [2]
U	The efficient score statistic [3]
V	Variance [4]
V_t	Contribution to the variance at time t [4]
V_{Trend}	Variance for logrank test for trend [5]
w_t	Weight at time t used in the calculation of the weighted Mantel–Haenszel test statistic [4]
W	The Wald statistic [6]
W_t	Relative weight at time t used in the calculation of the weighted Mantel–Haenszel test statistic [4]
x	Particular value of a variable [1]
	Indicator variable, taking values of 0 and 1 only [6]
z	The z-test, i.e. the ratio of an estimate to its SE [1]
$z_{1-\alpha/2}$	Value of the standardised normal deviate corresponding to a two-tailed area $1 - \alpha$ [1]
z(t)	Time-dependent covariate [8]

Index

Note: Figures and Tables are indicated by *italic page numbers*. 'p.h.' is abbreviation of 'proportional hazards'.